Praise for *Spotting Danger Before It Spots Your Kids* . . .

Gary's latest book, *Spotting Danger Before It Spots Your Kids,* is an amazing piece of work that can prepare your children for the unexpected dangers they may one-day face. Given that there is an epidemic of child sex trafficking right here in the United States, our children need to be educated about the importance of situational awareness, but parents and caregivers need to provide that education in a manner that won't completely terrify them. This book does an incredible job of giving adults the tools they need to do just that. Gary sets forth lessons that instill the basics of situational awareness in a way that is fun and engaging for both adults and kids. If there is a child in your life who you care about, please read this book.

—Craig Sawyer, founder of "Veterans for Child Rescue,"
former Navy SEAL, DEVGRU sniper

Many parents today believe that protecting their children from the dangers inherent in our society means avoiding sensitive issues and keeping their children locked away in a protective bubble. *Spotting Danger Before It Spots Your Kids* breaks you out of this mindset and shows you what children need to know if they are to navigate the uncertainties of the modern world. This book is a must-read for all new parents and young adults going off to high school or away to college.

—Joseph Koury, thirty-year veteran,
Special Operations soldier

When parents, especially mothers, attend my trainings, the number-one question I get asked is, "How do I teach my kids situational awareness without scaring them?" After reading Gary's book, I now have a resource I can recommend with complete confidence. Gary has taken all his knowledge and years of experience with the Federal Air Marshals and created a comprehensive and relatable step-by-step guide for building situational awareness skills in children. He shares stories of his own children's quick thinking, as well as heroic tales of children who knew what to do in an emergency situation; these stories offer parents positive examples of the importance of building these skills. Gary expertly identifies age-appropriate games that can be played by anyone and explains how they build lifesaving skills in children. This book is a must-read for every parent!

—Kelly Sayre, founder and president of The Diamond
Arrow Group, expert instructor in Situational Awareness
Training for Women, EAP consultant

T0126190

Spotting Danger Before It Spots Your Kids is a must for all parents. Not only does Gary give you everything you need to keep your family safe, he imparts years' worth of instructional experience. Gary shows you the tricks of the instructional trade and helps you relay this extremely important information. This book is not designed to instill fear. In fact, it will probably help the entire family to sleep better at night.

—Billy Williams, U.S. Department of Homeland Security supervisor, Counterterrorism and Explosives Training Section

As a former homicide and juvenile crimes detective sergeant, I can attest to the horrific dangers in the world we live in today. I know that if the victims of the crimes I investigated had had the tools contained in this book, they might still be alive. As a senior executive in law enforcement, I can confirm that there are grave dangers all around us. Most people are unaware of and often ill-equipped to survive these dangers. Gary is an expert in this field and teaches essential life-saving principles that are easy to learn and implement.

—Dana Chong Tim, government executive, former homicide and juvenile crimes detective-sergeant

In this book, Gary applies his expertise on situational awareness to issues unique to children, and does it in a completely entertaining way. This will be your go-to guidebook for creating real security for your family.

—Kelly D. Venden, retired Army Special Operations, federal law enforcement, owner of Criterion Tactical, LLC

Spotting Danger Before It Spots Your Kids: Teaching Children Situational Awareness to Stay Safe is one of those must-have parenting books. Gary Quesenberry is one of the premier experts in threat detection and situational awareness in the world. His vast experience makes him extremely qualified to offer his insights into any topic involving safety and security. He is also a proud husband and father who has put into practice the same techniques and methods while raising his own children. They are tested and proven. This is a fun and interactive book that helps kids figure out that they can have some level of control in their own lives and, more importantly, have the confidence that comes from knowing how to be safe and secure in any environment. It's a must for every bookshelf in America.

—Matt Cubbler, U.S. Army intelligence veteran, twenty-seven-year career law enforcement officer, former Special Agent with the U.S. Federal Air Marshal Service, author, speaker, host of the "Two Dates and a Dash Podcast"

I teach situational awareness, firearms courses, and instructor-level courses. I thought I was doing a pretty good job of passing on situational awareness skills to my children and grandchildren, but after reading this book, I have learned some things to up my game.

This is an excellent resource for parents and grandparents to help kids learn to be more situationally aware, listen to their gut instinct, be wise to the mood of their environment, and plan ahead for when things don't turn out to be all rainbows and unicorns. Plan on reading this book more than once because it is packed with great information!

—Dawn Dolpp, certified firearms instructor
and training counselor

This second book in Gary's situational awareness series is must-read primer for all parents who want to keep their children safe in the dangerous world we live in. Purchase this book, and you will learn from one of the best.

—Maureen Sangiorgio, award-winning writer,
NRA-certified firearms instructor/RSO

This book is truly eye opening! I deeply admire Gary's openness and honesty in sharing his family's own personal security scare. His story about having someone threaten his family's safety while he was away serving our country as the tip of the spear for Homeland Security operations really connected with me as a retired law enforcement officer. It clearly illustrated the all-too-common tendency to switch on our heightened awareness when needed and inadvertently switch it off when we are home with our loved ones. This book will make every parent take a step back and see the bigger picture and how it affects their family. I was a big fan of Gary's first book in this series, and this second book should be required reading for any parent out there.

—Trampas Swanson, firearms instructor/training counselor, deputy editor of *Private Military Contractor International* magazine, retired law enforcement officer

A brief, practical manual for parents and caregivers who want to help children identify and safely respond to dangerous situations.

A detailed but mostly straightforward kids-safety guide.

—*Kirkus Reviews*

SPOTTING DANGER BEFORE IT SPOTS YOUR KIDS

SPOTTING DANGER BEFORE IT SPOTS YOUR KIDS

Teaching Situational Awareness To Keep Children Safe

GARY QUESENBERRY
Federal Air Marshal (Ret.)

FOREWORD BY LOREN W. CHRISTENSEN

YMAA Publication Center
Wolfeboro, NH USA

YMAA Publication Center, Inc.
PO Box 480
Wolfeboro, New Hampshire 03894
1-800-669-8892 • info@ymaa.com • www.ymaa.com

ISBN: 9781594398117 (print) • ISBN: 9781594398124 (ebook)

Managing Editor: Doran Hunter
Cover design: Axie Breen
This book typeset in Sabon and Midiet

20210501

Images by Shutterstock unless otherwise noted

Publisher's Cataloging in Publication

Names: Quesenberry, Gary, author.

Title: Spotting danger before it spots your kids / Gary Quesenberry.

Description: Wolfeboro, NH USA : YMAA Publication Center, [2021] | "Teaching situational
          awareness to keep children safe."--Cover. | Includes bibliographical references and
          index.

Identifiers: ISBN: 9781594398117 (print) | 9781594398124 (ebook) | LCCN: 2021931531

Subjects: LCSH: Situational awareness--Safety measure--Parent participation. | Safety education--
          Parent participation. | Self-defense for children. | Self-protective behavior. |
          Self-preser- vation. | Self-defense for children--Psychological aspects. | Instinct. |
          Crime prevention --Psychological aspects. | Victims of crimes--Psychology. |
          Violence--Prevention. | Children-- Crimes against--Prevention. | BISAC: FAMILY
          & RELATIONSHIPS / Life Stages / School Age. | HEALTH & FITNESS / Safety. |
          SOCIAL SCIENCE / Violence in Society. | SPORTS & RECREATION / Martial
          Arts / General.

Classification: LCC: BF697.5.S45 Q471 2021 | DDC: 155.9/1--dc23

Note to Readers
Some identifying details have been changed to protect the privacy of individuals as well as the techniques and tactics employed by the Federal Air Marshal Service.

The authors and publisher of the material are NOT RESPONSIBLE in any manner whatsoever for any injury which may occur through reading or following the instructions in this manual.

The activities physical or otherwise, described in this manual may be too strenuous or dangerous for some people, and the reader(s) should consult a physician before engaging in them.

Warning: While self-defense is legal, fighting is illegal. If you don't know the difference you'll go to jail because you aren't defending yourself. You are fighting—or worse. Readers are encouraged to be aware of all appropriate local and national laws relating to self-defense, reasonable force, and the use of weaponry, and act in accordance with all applicable laws at all times. Understand that while legal definitions and interpretations are generally uniform, there are small—but very important—differences from state to state and even city to city. You need to know these differences. Neither the authors nor the publisher assumes any responsibility for the use or misuse of information contained in this book.

Nothing in this document constitutes a legal opinion nor should any of its contents be treated as such. While the authors believe that everything herein is accurate, any questions regarding specific self-defense situations, legal liability, and/or interpretation of federal, state, or local laws should always be addressed by an attorney at law.

When it comes to martial arts, self-defense, and related topics, no text, no matter how well written, can substitute for professional, hands-on instruction. **These materials should be used for academic study only.**

Printed in Canada.

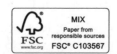

For Josh, Elda, and Emily
My pride and joy

Contents

Foreword
by Loren W. Christensen

I JOINED THE PORTLAND (OREGON) POLICE BUREAU shortly after returning from serving a year with the military police in Vietnam. Besides my regular duties as a patrol officer in Portland, I also taught self-defense to police officers at the bureau and situational awareness to citizens.

Outside of police work, I ran a martial arts school where I taught three fighting arts and always emphasized techniques to avoid conflict. I also wrote magazine pieces on alertness and awareness and, in time, I had mastered the subjects.

Or so I thought.

From 1988 through 1993, I worked in the police bureau's Gang Enforcement Team as an intelligence officer specializing in white supremacist gangs and hate crimes. I was also the media spokesman for the gang unit concerning racist skinheads. As such, I spoke to television, radio, and newspapers virtually every week. As a result, people recognized me on the street.

At one point, we learned through informants that at least one of the many skinhead gangs had compiled a hit list with my name at the top. I was an easy pick to kill because my name and face were continually in the public eye. Also on the list was a description of my private car, the type of firearm I carried, and the name of the school my two older children attended.

One blistering hot August day, my youngest daughter and I spent several hours enjoying a farmers' market set up in a downtown park. Wilted and sun-scorched, we left in the late afternoon to head home, wanting only to shower and lounge in front of the air conditioning. Almost home, we remembered we hadn't shopped for groceries yet. We stopped at a supermarket and slogged along like zombies through the aisles with a cart.

The next day after our grocery-buying stop, one of the gang unit's detectives stopped by my desk and asked if I had been shopping the day before at Safeway on 82nd with a girl about twelve years old. When I told him I had, he said, "It's a good thing you're sitting down."

The detective's informant had called him and said she had been shopping the day before when, as she put it, "I saw that cop who is on television walk past the end of her aisle with a young girl. Two skinheads who were in my row filling their cart with beer saw him too."

She heard one of them say to the other, "Hey, Officer Christensen just walked by with a kid. Let's do him in the parking lot." She heard the other skinhead say, "That must be his daughter; we'll kill her too."

She said the gang members pushed their cart to the end of the aisle to see where I had gone. When she saw us leave with our bags and the skinheads start to follow, she deliberately rammed her grocery cart into theirs with enough force to knock theirs over onto its side, spilling and breaking several beers. My daughter and I left the store, oblivious to the incident.

I was shocked to hear about the aborted hit and forever grateful to the woman who created a distraction. That my child was with me— well, there are no words to describe my anger.

I kept asking myself how I missed it all. Were the skinheads ever in my line of sight? If so, were they wearing the usual flight jackets, black work pants, and "Doc Marten" boots? They must have been if the woman recognized them as skins. So how did I miss them and the overturned grocery cart commotion?

I could tell myself they had not been where I could see them, and the grocery cart ramming had occurred after we were through checkout, but the one thing I know for sure is this—I wasn't alert in the store that afternoon. We were hot, exhausted, and frustrated that we had to buy groceries. We just wanted to get home. Nothing else mattered. Poor excuses? Yes, they are.

How disastrous it could have been if that woman hadn't been situationally aware that day to save my daughter and the guy who taught the subject to others.

Unfortunately, as a police officer, I investigated cases where there was no one to help the young victims. I'll spare you the details, but I will say this. The material in this book would have saved lives and psychological trauma.

Many have written and taught situational awareness for cops, martial artists, women, night workers, and other people in vulnerable occupations. But Gary Quesenberry's *Spotting Danger Before It Spots Your Kids* is unique because it's written for children, "our best hope for the future," as he says.

The book is also different from others because Gary has made the subject highly readable. Too many authors and instructors seem to try to present situational awareness as more complicated than it needs to be. Not Gary. His writing is immediately understandable, his analysis sound, and most importantly, his suggestions are easy to implement—right now.

Chapter One: The Parent's Role begins with the basics of situational awareness: 1) establishing a baseline of behavior within your given environment; 2) being able to spot actions that fall outside of that set baseline; and 3) developing plans for avoidance or escape based on what you see. These are the meat and potatoes of the entire program. Additionally, Gary tells parents to avoid teaching with fear. Brilliant! As a uniformed cop, I had so many parents point at me and say to their children that I would put them in jail if they didn't start behaving. Scaring kids doesn't work.

Chapter Two: How Children Learn New Tasks shows parents how their kids discover through three mediums: visual, auditory, and tactile. He offers several techniques for each one that help kids absorb and retain information.

Chapter Three: Teaching the Basics. Ask any top athlete, artist, musician, and rock climber what the essential element in their activity is, and they will answer—the basics. The same is true with personal safety.

Chapter Four: Game Night is about teaching children with games. Of the many Gary discusses, I especially liked "Drive [or walk] us home." With this one, the child provides directions back home to the parent, whether driving or walking. Be sure to include routes that pass police stations, firehouses, and hospitals.

Chapter Five, Situational Awareness for Children, introduces the core objectives of the program. Gary does an outstanding job of breaking down the four objectives without instilling fear.

Chapter Six: Give Your Children Options. In the first five chapters, Gary teaches the key elements that keep kids safe. In this one, he teaches four response options and how each one applies to various situations.

Chapter Seven: Common Encounters looks at situations in which kids are likely to find themselves, such as separation, interaction with strangers, and school shootings.

Chapter Eight: The "What If" Game. I played this many times with my children when they were growing up. I still do it sometimes when I'm out with one of them. I even do it with my wife, who has trained in the martial arts since 1996 and has black belts in two fighting systems. Refresher questions are a good thing at any age, including quizzing yourself.

Chapter Nine: Working Together. In this last chapter, Gary Quesenberry discusses how to work with children of different ages.

Spotting Danger Before It Spots Your Kids is, without question, the best book on the subject. It's easy to read, information-packed, well organized, and designed for quick reference.

Get it for your family and gift it to another parent.

Introduction

"It is not what you do for your children, but what you have taught them
to do for themselves, that will make them successful human beings."
—ANN LANDERS

LIKE ANY PARENT, I feel that children are our best hope for the future.
We commit our lives to giving them everything they need so we can
one day turn them loose in the world to flourish and grow. We want
them to have happy and healthy lives so maybe one day they can
experience the pleasure of loving and raising children of their own.
Regardless of how scary the thought of one day sending your children
out into the world may be, we need to prepare them in every way possible. That includes preparing them for the dangers they may one day
face. Nelson Mandela once said, "History will judge us by the difference we make in the everyday lives of children." I wholeheartedly
believe that to be true and feel that the most significant thing we can
do for our children is to give them a feeling of safety and security. As
parents, grandparents, uncles, and aunts, it's up to us to create an
environment where they will experience those feelings, but we also
have to teach them how to be self-sufficient. Their future success will

depend on their ability to interact with their surroundings and make sound decisions based on what they see. These same two concepts will also be what keeps them safe and free from harm as they start to become more independent.

According to healthychildren.org, children between the ages of four and six are beginning to seek their independence, form real friendships, and feel the need to perform more complex tasks on their own. At this age, it's also important for parents to start assigning more responsibility to their children. Aside from the ordinary duties of cleaning their rooms and brushing their teeth before bed, it's time to start thinking of ways we can teach them to look out for themselves. One effective way of beginning this process is by informing your children about situational awareness and the critical role it plays in their personal safety. Most adults have a basic understanding of situational awareness and what that means. My definition of situational awareness is this: the ability to identify and process environmental cues to accurately predict the actions of others. As adults, we do this daily without giving it much thought. We do it during our commutes to work, in grocery store checkout lines, and in parking lots. We are continually taking in information and using what we see to make decisions. The question is, how do we best take the basic concepts of situational awareness and present them to our children? On the surface, this may not seem like a very pressing issue. Our children's safety is our responsibility, and as parents, we try to be present and available as much as humanly possible, but what happens when we can't be there? What do our children need to know about spotting danger and keeping themselves safe?

For the past twenty-eight years, I've either been in the military or working in federal law enforcement. As a federal air marshal, it was my job to blend into my surroundings and pay close attention to what was going on around me. Situational awareness, planning, and preparation became second nature, and the process of predicting the actions of others became almost intuitive. This isn't a superpower or some secret skill reserved only for those working in high-speed counterterror jobs. Awareness is something that everyone possesses to one degree or another. Some of what we know about others is instinctive; the rest is based on observable patterns of behavior and what those behaviors mean in the context of a given situation. It wasn't until a terrifying incident involving my own family that I realized how vital these skills were to everyone, especially children. (Readers of my first book will recall this story.)

The incident happened back in 2003. I was working as a federal air marshal in Las Vegas, Nevada. A man identifying himself as Gary Quesenberry called my children's elementary school and told the attendance officer he would be coming by to pick the kids up early. He said that because he worked for the government, he was being reassigned to a new office, and the children would not be returning. The caller knew my name, the names of my children, and that I worked for the government. To me, this was an apparent attempt by someone to get at my family. Luckily, my wife regularly volunteered at the school and had stopped by early that day. She knew that I was away at work that night and quickly alerted the police to the situation. No one ever showed up, and we believe the added police presence at the school scared off the would-be kidnapper. The jobs I've held over the years always left me open to predatorial targeting. Still, we've constantly cautioned our children against strangers and how they should react if someone unfamiliar approached them. Hopefully the school's system of identification would have eliminated any chance of someone removing the kids that day. I had no idea what had happened to cause this, but it was clear to me that changes had to be made, not only in the way my wife and I did things but also in what we taught our children about personal safety. It was time to get serious about hardening our defenses and the first place we started was with situational awareness.

Situational awareness consists of three parts:

1. Establishing a baseline of behavior within your given environment
2. Being able to spot actions that fall outside of that set baseline
3. Developing plans for avoidance or escape based on what you see.

We're going to get deeper into those things later, but it's important to remember that those three factors do not change depending on your age. Whether you're eight years old or eighty, those are the three elements of situational awareness that can save your life. The question becomes, how do we teach those three things to children in a way they'll appreciate and understand?

As my wife and I began teaching our kids about situational awareness, one thing became glaringly obvious: the old model of "stranger danger" just didn't work. I wanted my children to be friendly and engaging, and by teaching them that all strangers are dangerous, we were actually instilling an unnecessary amount of fear in them. According to the National Center for Missing and Exploited Children, roughly 800,000 children are reported missing each year in the United States. That's approximately 2,200 per day. Of those, there are 115 "stranger abduction" cases, which accounts for less than one percent of the annual total. The truth is, not all strangers are dangerous; they may be parents themselves, or grandparents, teachers, pastors, or nurses. Regardless of who they are, the vast majority of people are reasonable, law-abiding citizens who would go out of their way to help a child in need. Children can be entirely crippled by fear, and the last thing my wife and I wanted as parents were to be the source of that fear. We wanted our kids to be confident and outgoing, but what was the best way to allow them to retain those social traits and still teach them about the potential for danger and the importance of personal safety? That question led me to take a closer look at the federal air marshal's program of situational awareness and how the things I'd learned over the course of my career could be adapted to, and successfully taught to, children.

To simplify the process of teaching situational awareness to children, I've broken this book down into three separate phases.

1. **What parents need to know.** It's imperative that adults have a firm grip on the fundamentals of situational awareness and how they impact personal safety. Phase one will serve as a refresher for the concepts I've detailed in *Spotting Danger Before It Spots You*, book one of the Heads Up series and will be the jumping off point for the techniques you'll pass along to your children.

2. **What kids need to know.** This is where we take a closer look at the basics of awareness from the child's perspective and start laying the groundwork for a more progressive situational awareness program.

3. **Teaching and reinforcing the specific aspects of situational awareness.** This is where the real work begins. In this phase, adults and children will work together to build upon the foundations laid in phase two. The skills that your child has developed can now be utilized in specific training points that emphasize the importance of situational awareness and ensure that your child understands their full range of options during a dangerous encounter.

In the appendix, I've included an easy-to-follow checklist. This roadmap to situational awareness will help you stay on track and monitor you and your child's progress along their journey to personal safety.

As I mentioned above, we'll be revisiting some of the concepts covered in the first book. I felt that in certain chapters it was necessary to refresh the reader's memory on some key components of situational awareness. In other cases, I worked under the assumption that the reader may not have read the first book at all. In either case I've made an attempt to keep repetitive material brief and relevant to the topics being discussed.

The basics of situational awareness aren't overly complicated. I found early on that the fundamental elements of awareness, such as memory, comprehension, critical thinking, and decision-making, could be easily taught and reinforced through simple games. Once those skill sets are in place, it becomes much easier to advance children into the more focused aspects of awareness.

Before we begin, I'd like to make one thing clear. I'm not a child psychologist. I'm simply a parent who, through the course of a career as a federal air marshal, has learned how to observe and read people's actions without drawing undue attention to himself. What I give to you here is a simple and effective method for presenting your children with the building blocks of situational awareness—a road map to help you guide them along their journey to personal safety. As with any new skill, these things take time and practice. If you stick with it and keep the process fun and engaging, you'll start to notice a big difference in the way your child interacts with their surroundings. You'll see them begin to identify and differentiate between normal and abnormal behaviors in various settings. You'll also see how these newfound skills improve their spatial awareness and ability to think critically about their environment. Eventually, you'll feel more confident in the fact that, even when alone, your child can spot dangerous situations before they happen, act independently, and communicate effectively with those around them. These are potentially life-saving skills, but the process of learning them can also serve as a means for quality family time. As I said in the beginning, our children are our best hope for the future. We're obligated to give them everything they need to stay happy and safe. Their situational awareness plays a big role in that, so let's get started.

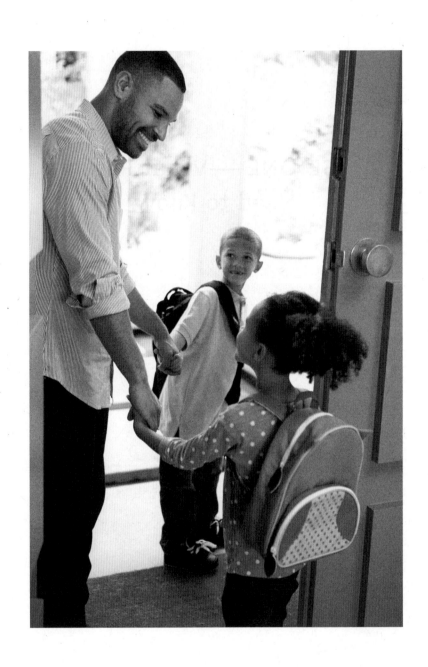

PHASE ONE—What Parents Need to Know

1

The Parent's Role

"It's a great mistake, I think, to put children off with falsehoods and nonsense when their growing powers of observation and discrimination excite in them a desire to know about things."

—ANNE SULLIVAN

AS PARENTS, WE HAVE a great responsibility. Not only are we responsible for the safety and wellbeing of our children, but we are also tasked with guiding them along the path to independence. We were all kids at some point. As adults, it becomes harder to connect with the feelings we had as children. We tend to look back at our childhood experiences with an adult perspective, and in doing so we wonder how we could have ever been so happily oblivious. What we need to remember is that the dangers young people face today are dramatically different than those we faced even a decade ago. Things change, and as the world becomes more challenging, we need to take the time to prepare our children. Not in a way that will scare them into staying locked up inside the house, but in a way that is fun, engaging, and will give them the best possible chance of ensuring their own wellbeing. This all starts by tapping into your child's greatest resource ... their imagination.

According to child psychologist Sally Goddard Blythe, director of The Institute for Neuro-Physiological Psychology, the importance of imagination in childhood development cannot be overstated. "Put simply, imagination is the ability to create visual images in the mind's eye, which allows us to explore all sorts of images and ideas without being constrained by the limits of the physical world. This is how children begin to develop problem-solving skills, coming up with new possibilities, new ways of seeing and being, which develop important faculties in critical thinking that will help the child throughout life." These elements of critical thinking and problem-solving are crucial to the development of situational awareness. It's up to us parents to tap into this well of imagination and use our children's natural curiosity to impart lessons that foster a sense of independence and security.

Adults have a unique opportunity. We can use our children's ability to imagine and create as a way to teach them about things they may not necessarily be interested in. I know from experience that talking to kids about safety and awareness isn't something that immediately gains their attention. Trying to broach these subjects in a way that holds your child's interest is challenging, to say the least, but to get them fully involved, you must have a thorough understanding of the topic yourself. Children learn by example. Whether you're aware of it or not, they watch every move you make, and they try to imitate the things they see you doing. From the way you walk, talk, and interact with others, your children are constantly evaluating you. It's essential that you use this knowledge to set a good example, but it's also a vital piece of the awareness puzzle. Your children's natural curiosity and capacity for observation are what we're going to focus on to build their situational awareness. They already have all the tools they need to develop these abilities and adapt them into their life; what's most important right now is that you, as the parent, have the tools you need. So let's start with the basics.

1.1 The Basics of Awareness

Your personal security is about much more than just your immediate circumstances. Real safety comes from being able to predict the actions of others through observation and planning. This is the heart and soul of situational awareness and takes place well before any physical encounter with danger. If you've read the first book in the Heads Up series, you should already have a pretty good grip on the basics of situational awareness and how specific techniques can be readily applied to help you identify the behaviors that accompany violent action. By identifying these behaviors early, you're giving yourself a head start on the decision-making process and, ideally, avoiding dangerous situations before they even occur. Building proper situational awareness begins with understanding the basic levels of awareness and how they affect your reactions.

Situational awareness can be separated into five levels. These levels of awareness are most commonly referred to as "Cooper's Colors." The Cooper color code system of awareness was developed by Marine Corps Lieutenant Colonel Jeff Cooper and includes five conditions, or colors, that represent a person's mental state as they go about their daily activities. These five levels explain the general ranges of situational awareness and the psychological states associated with each level.

1. **Condition White:** In this condition, a person is entirely relaxed and unaware of what's going on around them. For instance, someone walking along staring at their cell phone while listening to music through his or her headphones could be considered in condition white. They've effectively cut themselves off by blocking out all visual and auditory indicators they may receive from their surroundings. In the majority of cases, condition white is reserved for when you are asleep or when you find yourself in an environment that you assume to be completely free of threats, like your own home. Criminals generally target people they deem to be in condition white because their lack of awareness makes them look like easy prey. If you are ever attacked while in condition white, the chances of escape are severely diminished because your attacker will have caught you off guard. Your actions at that point will be completely reactionary.

2. **Condition Yellow:** This is a state of relaxed awareness and the condition that allows you to most effectively take in your surroundings. You appear to those around you to be entirely comfortable in your environment while paying close attention to the sights and sounds that surround you. This condition of awareness does not constitute a state of paranoia or hyper-vigilance. Instead, you've simply upped your awareness to a level that would prevent you from being caught off guard.

3. **Condition Orange:** At this stage, you have identified something that could be perceived as a threat, and you've narrowed your attention to that specific person or area. You quickly notice abnormal behaviors in others and shift your level of awareness to accommodate for those actions. This is also the stage where you begin to put together spontaneous plans, and the anticipation of action starts to elevate your heart rate. Once the perceived threat has passed, it's easy to relax and transition from condition orange back to yellow.

4. **Condition Red:** This is where you find yourself right before you act on your plans. In condition orange, you spotted a perceived threat and began the planning stages for an appropriate reaction. In condition red, the threat has materialized, and it's time to put those plans into action. This is where the heart rate becomes more elevated, and the fight, flight, or freeze responses are triggered. Your body prepares itself for confrontation, and the adrenaline starts pumping into your system. Condition red is where your level of training has a significant impact on how the situation is resolved.

5. **Condition Black:** Condition black is much like condition white in that you do not want to find yourself there when the fight starts. Condition black is characterized by an excessively elevated heart rate (above 175 beats per minute) and a complete loss of cognitive ability. A person in condition black lacks the

power to process the information being taken in effectively and becomes utterly useless in terms of response.

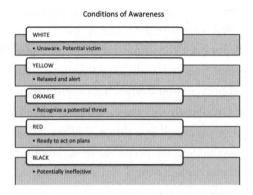

Conditions of Awareness

WHITE
• Unaware. Potential victim

YELLOW
• Relaxed and alert

ORANGE
• Recognize a potential threat

RED
• Ready to act on plans

BLACK
• Potentially ineffective

When it comes to maintaining proper situational awareness, you always want to stay in condition yellow. You want to be in that casual yet observant state that allows you to take in as much information as possible without completely stressing yourself out. That brings us to the next piece of the awareness puzzle, which requires planning. If you're in condition yellow and spot something you perceive as a possible threat, you have to start making plans for a reasonable response to that threat; any time that happens, it triggers what is known as the OODA loop.

Originally developed by Air Force fighter pilot John Boyd, the OODA loop is designed to help you quickly assess a situation and create a plan of action. The loop consists of four stages: Observe, Orient, Decide, and Act. Here's what happens in each step:

1. **Observe:** You make an observation about something happening within your environment.
2. **Orient:** This involves an understanding of your environmental norms to help better identify potential problems.
3. **Decide:** You develop a plan of action based on information gathered during the orientation phase.
4. **Act:** You put that plan into action.

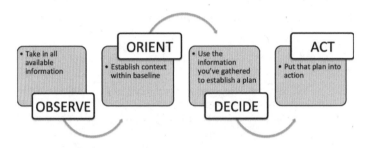

It's often said that action is quicker than reaction, but more accurately, it's unanticipated action that catches you off guard and slows down your response time. By maintaining a condition yellow level of awareness, you can more quickly identify threats to your personal safety and decrease your reactionary times by being forewarned of a potential problem. Most often, the OODA loop process takes from one to three seconds from observation to action. This space of time is commonly referred to as the reactionary gap and can be decreased with proper training and practice. Cooper's color system and the OODA loop are just two fundamental elements of situational awareness. They illustrate where your level of awareness should be at any given time, what physiological effects can be expected, and how those affect your decision-making and reaction times.

I often get asked what I feel is the most critical aspect of personal safety. People usually expect me to answer with something along the lines of "develop a winning mindset" or "seek training in some form of self-defense," but the answer is much more straightforward. The most important aspect of personal safety is something that's built into us naturally. It's an integral part of situational awareness. Still, few people ever take the time to listen to or develop it properly. It's our intuition. Author Gavin de Becker, who wrote the incredible book, *The Gift of Fear: Survival Signs That Protect Us*, once said that "intuition is always right in at least two important ways; it is always in response to something. It always has our best interest at heart." What most people refer to as intuition is actually a cognitive process. When we feel threatened, this cognitive process moves faster than we can possibly control or perceive. We often second-guess our gut feelings because we put much more trust in the logical step-by-step approach to thinking. Some of the signals our brain sends us to warn of danger we disregard as trivial and unimportant because it's too hard for us to connect the dots between what we see and the risk that lies ahead. We owe it to ourselves to pay closer attention to these "gut feelings." They're built into our DNA, and their sole purpose is to keep us safe from danger.

Imagine the following scenario: you're walking across a parking lot to your car with an armful of groceries. A kind stranger approaches you and offers to help. His sudden appearance startles you, and your first instinct is to refuse the offer and continue on. Still, the man seems charming enough, and he promises to just help you get your groceries into the trunk and move along. He is standing between you and your car, smiling politely, so you accept the offer. I know for a fact that some readers are screaming internally, "NOOOO! Do not let that man near you!" There are several indicators in this scenario that let us know this guy is up to no good. The sudden approach, the unsolicited promises to move along after he's helped you out, and the impeding of your movement. All of these indicators point to danger, and we'll cover more of these in greater detail later on, but the most important thing to take away from this is that the first instinct our fictional victim had was to refuse the offer for help. That "gut feeling" is intuition. It's your brain taking in all of the environmental indicators, detecting the possibility of danger, and overriding your rational mind to warn you of a threat to your safety.

Every animal on the planet is hardwired with instinct and intuition. Unfortunately, we humans are the only ones who think we're smarter than Mother Nature. We see the possibility of a threat, we sense danger, and we have all the tools we need to escape it, but instead of acting on our instincts, we try to rationalize its presence and explain it away. Intuition is an incredibly useful tool. It allows you to harness the powers of your subconscious mind to make judgments that can prevent bad people from getting too close to you, and it could quite possibly save your life. Always listen when intuition speaks to you.

These three things, Cooper's colors, the OODA loop, and intuition lay the foundation for the system of awareness that I teach. They'll help to guide your children along the path to awareness as well. Now that you're familiar with these fundamental concepts, it's time to move on to the more focused aspects of situational awareness. We'll start by establishing what is known as a behavioral baseline.

Any time you walk into a new environment, you need to ask yourself one question: "Is the feeling I get from this place a good feeling or a bad feeling?" If the feeling you get from a place or a person is a good one, then there's seldom a need to worry, but if you enter into a situation and immediately get a bad feeling, you need to stop yourself and take a closer look at things. What is happening around you that set those alarm bells off? The best way to identify those things is to have a firm understanding of behavioral baselines. Every person, place, or situation has a specific set of behaviors that are generally adhered to. If you walk into a supermarket, you have a pretty good idea of how the people there should be acting: pushing shopping carts, browsing aisles, and waiting patiently in checkout lines. That's the behavioral baseline for that particular space. If, however, someone in line began shouting loudly and threatening the other customers, that action would fall way outside of the established baseline. It's usually when we spot something that falls outside of the baseline that we tend to get those bad feelings. Before you walk into any given situation, it's a good idea to have a general understanding of what the common behaviors are for that area. If you're comfortable with your surroundings and the things that are happening around you, then it's time to begin an initial scan. The initial scan of an area is nothing more than a quick glance around to see if there are any particular people or actions that fall outside of the baseline. If you spot something that makes you uncomfortable, then it may be a good idea to just remove yourself from the situation, but if that isn't possible, it's time to start developing a plan of action. This could include a hasty escape or even confrontation, but it's imperative that you have those plans in place before it's time to act.

Understanding behavioral baselines, spotting baseline anomalies, and developing plans of action are what will serve as the starting point for what we teach our children about situational awareness. As I mentioned earlier, I feel that the old "stranger danger" model actually does more harm than good and serves no purpose other than building unwarranted fear in our children. We adults can sometimes be crippled by irrational fear as well. We need to be able to differentiate between the actions and encounters that actually pose a threat to our safety and our preconceived notions about other people. Understand that threats can come from anywhere at any time. I spent six years working in a federal prison, and if I learned one thing, it's that dangerous people seldom fit a stereotypical image. Some of the most dangerous men I've ever met were well under six feet tall and only weighed about 160 pounds. They looked meek and unassuming as opposed to imposing and aggressive—the exact opposite of what I had previously imagined a dangerous person to look like. Learning to put aside your preconceived ideas about dangerous people is particularly important when you start talking to your children about safety. They need to be able to discern between perceived danger and the observable actions that actually accompany violence.

Now we're going to use what you know about your surroundings and the accompanying baseline behaviors to identify those observable actions, anticipate potential problems, and plan appropriate responses should one of those problems materialize.

Criminals are cunning, and they know how to stay hidden until it's time to strike, but they also tend to stick to patterns of behavior you can easily identify if you know what to look for. The process of watching for changes within your environment is known as a detailed scan. During the detailed scan, you're recognizing and collecting behavioral cues that help you to identify people in your area who may be up to no good. Here it's important to focus on those behaviors that are universal and apply to everyone regardless of age, race, sex, or background. These identifiable behaviors are known as "pre-incident indicators." Pre-incident indicators are common patterns of behavior that criminals tend to stick to and generally include the following:

- **Hidden hands:** The hands are what can kill you. Someone who is hiding their hands may also be concealing their intent to harm you.

- **Inexplicable presence:** Does the person who caught your attention have a reason for being where they are? Is their presence justified and their actions in alignment with the baseline behaviors of that area?

- **Target glancing:** Predators like to keep an eye on their prey, but in an attempt to avoid eye contact, they will continually glance at and away from their intended victim.

- **A sudden change of movement:** If you feel that you are being followed and suddenly change your direction of travel, keep an eye on the people around you. If someone inexplicably changes their direction of travel to match yours, you could be their target.

- **Inappropriate clothing:** Someone who is wearing more clothing than is appropriate may be trying to hide something.

- **Seeking a position of advantage:** Predators like to keep the upper hand. In an attempt to gain dominance, they will try to maneuver themselves into positions where they know they will have the tactical advantage. For example, an aggressor may try to back you into a corner where escape would be more difficult, or purposely block an exit.

- **Impeding your movement:** If someone inexplicably blocks your movement in a particular direction, there's a pretty good chance they're trying to funnel you into a position of disadvantage.

- **Unsolicited attempts at conversation:** If someone you are unfamiliar with approaches you and makes an attempt at unwanted small talk, take a very close look at your situation. Are you in a position of disadvantage? Are there other people in the area? Has this person shown other pre-incident indicators that lead you to believe they have bad intentions? Attempts at small talk are often the predator's last move before the attack.

These are just a handful of pre-incident indicators that are common in predatory behavior. One of these behaviors can be easily over-looked. Two could be considered coincidental, but once someone steps outside of the established baseline and has exhibited at least three abnormal behaviors, it's safe to assume that that person is up to no good. In law enforcement, this is known as the "Rule of Three" because it rises above the level of coincidence and moves into the realm of suspicious behavior.

Aside from the pre-incident indicators we just covered, there are also specific uncontrollable physiological reactions to stress that often act as precursors to violence. Here are a few of the more common physiological indicators that someone is ready to strike.

- **Heavier than usual breathing:** When someone is under stress, his or her respiratory system is immediately affected. They begin to breathe heavier or take sudden deep breaths to help distribute oxygen-rich blood to their extremities just in case they feel the need to fight or flee. Someone who intends to assault another person may appear to be breathing heavier than normal as they "psych themselves up" for the attack.
- **Appearing tense:** When we're placed under stress, our muscles naturally tense up to help protect us from injury and pain.
- **Posturing:** People who feel threatened will naturally attempt to make themselves appear bigger. They'll puff out their chest, spread their arms, or become louder to ward off any potential threats or intimidate their intended victims.
- **Pupil dilation:** This is when a person's pupils appear larger and is often associated with fear and anger. Usually, a person's pupils

are two to five millimeters in diameter but can dilate to as large as nine millimeters when they feel threatened. This can take place within the space of a second and is a sure-fire way to gauge a person's emotional state, but it also requires you to be dangerously close to the subject.

- **Excessive sweating:** Sweating is a natural reaction to fear and stress regardless of the outside temperature.

These five items are not all-inclusive, but they offer a pretty good sample of normal physiological reactions to stressful circumstances. When paired with the known pre-incident indicators, they can quickly help identify someone who poses a real threat to your safety. This, in turn, can help you accurately anticipate their actions and plan your responses appropriately.

So there you have it. The basics of how situational awareness plays a role in preserving your personal safety. At this point you should fully understand:

1. How to establish a baseline of behavior within your given environment.
2. How to spot actions that fall outside of that set baseline and are in the realm of suspicious behavior.
3. How to use that information to circumvent dangerous situations and ensure your own safety.

Now you have to ask yourself, how do I present this same information to my children in a way that will keep them engaged and eager to learn? We're going to answer that question in chapter 2, but there are a couple of other relevant topics I feel should be addressed before we move on.

1.2 The Pros and Cons of Technology

We live in an unbelievable age. We walk around with devices in our pockets that allow us to communicate with people on the other side of the planet, predict the weather, and answer just about any question you ask it. Some of our cars can now drive and park themselves, and we have cameras in the farthest reaches of outer space. Technology is advancing in ways I couldn't even imagine just ten years ago. All of these advancements are designed to make our lives easier, but I often warn others against letting technology take over their lives to the point that it becomes a threat to personal safety. I don't mean this in the sense that artificial intelligence will one day take over and enslave the human race; I mean that we can sometimes let our connection to technology keep us from focusing on the more common tasks we should be performing. Take driving for instance. Driving is a task that requires all of our mental faculties to not only pay attention to what we're doing but to pay attention to the other drivers on the road as well. There is no room for multitasking when it comes to driving. The National Safety Council reports that cell phone use while driving leads to 1.6 million crashes each year. Nearly 390,000 injuries occur each year from accidents caused by texting while driving, and one out of every four car accidents in the United States is caused by texting and driving. These are staggering numbers that illustrate how our reliance on technology can sometimes cause serious problems. Our situational awareness when driving is obviously critical, but what about awareness when you're just walking along the sidewalk? Again, when we're talking about preserving your personal safety, this is no time for multitasking.

An entire book could be written about the dangers of online predators who target children using technological means. As parents, we must familiarize ourselves with these dangers and do everything we can to protect our kids against predatory targeting. For the purpose of this book, however, I'm going to limit the discussion about children and technology to how overuse can have a negative impact on their situational awareness. According to a 2017 study conducted by Common Sense Media, American children ages five to eight spend nearly three hours on their screens daily. Between the ages of eight and twelve, they spend roughly four hours and forty-four minutes a day on mobile devices. Once they hit their teens, that number increases to seven hours and twenty-two minutes daily. That's a lot of screen time, and let's face it, some of the time our children spend on mobile devices should actually be spent paying attention to their surroundings. The distraction that's caused by the technology we use can be so overpowering that it can sometimes lead to serious bodily injury. As a federal air marshal, I've spent an enormous amount of time transiting through airports. I've watched children and teens get so drawn into their iPads and phones that they've fallen down escalators, walked into glass doors, and become completely separated from their parents. I'm not saying that technology is terrible, but it's important that we teach our children when its use is appropriate and when their focus should be on what's happening around them. We need to keep this in mind when we begin to talk to our children about situational awareness. Our kids learn by what they see, and if they see you constantly attached to your phone, this will be the behavior they consider normal. We have to pick our heads up and lead by example if we really want to help our children understand and interact with their surroundings.

1.3 Avoid Teaching Fear

Fear can have crippling effects on both children and adults. Most people have some sort of irrational phobia; maybe it's spiders, tight spaces, dogs, or just a general fear of other people. What you have to remember is that most fears are entirely illogical and based primarily on our preconceived notions about people and things. Some of these fears we develop through past experiences; for example, maybe a dog bit someone when they were young, and now that fear of dogs has followed them into adulthood. Another way we can develop irrational fears is by inheriting them. Children learn from example, and if they see an adult in their lives exhibit a fear such as a fear of heights, then the child is much more likely to develop that fear themselves. Dr. Francine Rosenberg, a clinical psychologist and anxiety specialist at

Morristown Memorial Hospital in New Jersey, said, "This learning occurs through parents' verbal and nonverbal cues to their children." The best way to prevent children from inheriting their fears or phobias is for adults to acknowledge and evaluate the validity of their own fears. Once we can confront and control our anxieties, it becomes easier to help our children navigate their own. Here are four ways I've found to help guide my kids through their own fears.

1. **Take your child's fear seriously:** Although some fears may be irrational, they are all very real and can have devastating effects on our mental state. The fear of interpersonal human aggression can be very frightening and cause us to avoid interacting with others. The fear of financial loss, the death of a loved one, or sickness are all genuine and relevant fears. As adults, we deal with these fears as best we can, and we try not to let the effects of this fear spread to our children. In doing so, we can sometimes forget that our child's fear of "the monster under the bed," although irrational to us, is just as real and scary as the fears you have as an adult. Allow your child to express their concerns without judgment. Acknowledge that the fear exists, and then you can begin to work through it together.

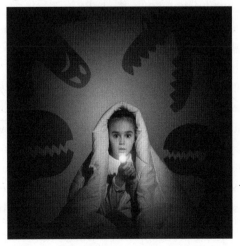

2. **Work together:** "Once you've offered reassurance, it's important to move on quickly," says Dr. Rachel Busman, a clinical psychologist at the Child Mind Institute. "We don't want to dwell on offering comfort around the scary thing, because even that can become reinforcing and take on a life of its own." Instead, start talking about how you'll work together to help your child start feeling braver and get to the point where they're able to manage the fear on their own.

3. **Give your child control:** Both of my daughters used to have an issue with going to bed on their own. Both wanted me or their mom to stay in their rooms, sing, tell stories, play … anything but sleep. Eventually, we had do develop a plan to control their fear of being alone at night so that we could all get to bed at a reasonable hour. The idea was to get them to put themselves to bed by the end of the month, and it went something like this:

- Week 1: Business as usual, but we started talking to the girls more seriously about why it was important for them to start putting themselves to bed.
- Week 2: We would read one story, sing one song together, and then mommy or daddy would tuck them in, turn off the lights, and be right down the hall.
- Week 3: We would read one story or sing one song (not both). Then, the girls could turn off the lights themselves, and we would all go to bed.
- Week 4: We could read and sing before bedtime, but once the girls were in their rooms, it was their responsibility to turn their lights out and put themselves to bed. By slowly allowing our girls to take more control over their own routine, they began to feel more independent and less fearful. You have to remember that this exchange of control takes time and won't always be easy. But try to be encouraging. Compliment your

children on their bravery and let them know that you're
proud of them every chance you get.

4. **Don't use fear as a tool:** One thing that's always bothered me is
when I see adults using fear to control children. Fear of abstract
concepts like "the boogeyman" are perfectly normal, but parents
often use authoritative figures to scare and regulate their
children's behavior. A good friend of mine used to be a uniformed police officer in Las Vegas. He once told me a story that
perfectly illustrates how using fear to manage your children is a
bad idea. Like most police officers, he would take overtime
shifts wherever he could to help make ends meet. One night he
was working in a local shopping center where a woman entered
with a very unruly young son. When the woman realized that
she wouldn't be able to control her child, she pointed at my
friend and said, "Do you see that police officer over there? If
you don't behave, I'm going to have him arrest you and take
you to jail. Is that what you want?" My friend approached the
woman, and calmly informed her that what she was doing was
counterproductive. She may have felt that what she said would
help control her child, but what she had actually done was
instill in him an irrational fear of police officers. Now, if he ever
found himself in trouble or separated from his mother, his
natural inclination would be to avoid the police officer as
opposed to seeking help. Author Gavin de Becker points out in
his amazing book, *Protecting the Gift, Keeping Children and
Teenagers Safe (and Parents Sane)* that when parents want to
underscore the importance of some given instruction, they often
attach some scary outcome to it: "Come right home; you don't
want to get kidnapped"; "Don't go there alone, remember
anyone could be a killer." These scare tactics don't work and can
only have two possible outcomes.

- It will work and the child will be afraid.
- It won't work and the parent will lose credibility.

The parent who loses credibility is not an effective teacher. How effective is it to tell your child that sitting too close to the television will cause them to go blind, when they know full well that it won't? If your child thinks all parental warnings are just a litany of outlandish claims, they will be less likely to believe any of them.

Parents have to pay close attention to the fears of their children, and in most cases, we have the tools we need to help them work through their anxieties. On the other hand, if your child's fears are persistent, overly intense, or begin interfering with their daily life, it might be time to seek some outside help. According to The Child Mind Institute, signs that a fear may be something more include:

- Obsessive worrying: Your child fixates on the object of their fear, thinking or talking about it often, or even when the trigger isn't present. For example, becoming terribly anxious months before their next dentist visit.
- Fears that limit your child's ability to enjoy their life or participate in activities. For example, refusing to go on a class trip to the park because there might be dogs there.
- Panic attacks.
- Compulsive or disruptive behavior.
- Withdrawing from activities, school, or family.

If your child's fears seem like they might be something more serious, make an appointment to talk with a professional to see if more help is necessary.

About five years after my girls overcame their fear of being alone at night, I began working with them on various forms of self-defense. Situational awareness exercises, hand-to-hand defensive techniques, and firearms safety were just a few common topics in the Quesenberry house. Part of teaching your kids about the scarier aspects of life is to take the mystery out of it and even expose them to a little controlled fear once in a while to gauge their reactions to it. Be honest, we've all taken the opportunity to prank our kids with a good scare from time to time. I'm personally notorious for this. I clearly remember the night our little training sessions began to take hold, and things took a drastic turn for dear old Dad. I had recently accepted a position as the lead firearms instructor at the Federal Air Marshal Training Center in New Jersey. My daughters shared a room that had a large walk-in closet along the wall opposite their beds. One night my wife and I decided to watch *The Shining*. The girls wanted to watch it with us and simply wouldn't take no for an answer. Needless to say, when the movie was over, the girls were terrified. My wife and I quickly developed a plan to give them a good scare before bed, just to teach them a lesson. My wife kept the girls occupied in the living room while I acted like I was taking the dog out for a walk. Instead of taking the dog out, I quietly slipped into their room and hid in the big walk-in closet, waiting for my chance to scare them. My wife then sent them to bed, knowing that I was set and ready. As I listened at the closet door, I could hear the girls getting into their beds. Once I thought they were settled, I began growling and scratching at the door. I was so giddy at the opportunity to scare the bejesus out of them I could barely contain myself. I could hear the girls whispering to each other outside the door and shuffling around. In my mind's eye, I could imagine the girls jumping in bed with one another and pulling the covers up over their heads in fright. That's when I pounced. I swung the door open and screamed at the top of my lungs. But instead of two terrified little girls, I was met with a hastily built barricade behind which my oldest daughter Elda stood with a fully loaded Nerf gun pointed directly at my chest. She was in a perfect modified isosceles stance and her two-hand thumbs-forward grip was impeccable. She had her little sister Emily behind her ready to protect her at all costs. I had never been more proud! Not only had my baby girl controlled her fear, she also confronted it head-on.

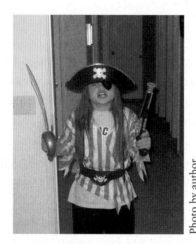

Elda the Defender.

I tell this story not to illustrate what a devious parent I can be, but to point out that children are fully capable of tackling fears on their own. They learn these skills through the actions they see us taking as adults and the lessons we provide them. Once we understand how important it is to set a good example by controlling our own fears, we can start working together with our children to help them master the skills they'll need to develop their situational awareness.

Kids in Action

Landon Clemmer Saves His Mom

Eleven-year-old Landon Clemmer lives in Chattanooga, Tennessee, and is being honored as a hero by local first responders. One evening while playing video games in his room, Landon heard a loud thud. He knew that his mother Heather was in the next room bathing his younger sister, so he decided it would be best to check on them. Landon knocked on the bathroom door and asked his mother if everything was okay, but she didn't respond. That's when he started hearing unfamiliar noises come from inside. He opened the door and immediately saw his mother's head slipping underwater. Local emergency medical services officials said his mother had a seizure and fell over into the bathtub. "My mom always taught me not to panic, so I just pulled her out and then called 911 when I realized she was having a seizure." He had recently witnessed his friend's mom have a seizure, so he knew that he needed to lay her on her side to prevent her from choking. "After a little bit, she got up. She wasn't talking; she was just walking through the halls," said Landon. Once emergency responders were inside the house, they started checking Heather's responsiveness. She recalled that "they started asking me questions like who is the president, how old are you, and I was completely blown away, I had no idea any of the answers." She said she felt like her mind was wiped clean. She only remembered waking up to paramedics in her driveway. Sabrina Johnson, a responding paramedic, said Landon did everything right that night.

"He did better than most adults would have done in that situation because a seizure is a scary thing. To see and then especially when you see your mom having one when she's never had one before, that's pretty scary." Landon told his mom he hopes to be a firefighter when he's older. His mom said, "It's like that's what he was made to do, he's there to handle stuff like that. He's very protective over me and his sister." Landon reacted calmly because that's what his mother had taught him, to remain composed and avoid panic. The lessons she had given him proved very valuable that night, and young Landon rose to the occasion. He was later presented with a certificate of appreciation from Hamilton County EMS officials during a ceremony to honor his bravery.[1]

---

1 "Boy, 11, Honored after Quick Action Saves Mom's Life," https://abc7chi-cago.com/boy-11-honored-after-quick-action-saves-mom/5470338/.

Exercise

Find something that your child may be frightened of, something like going to bed alone, playing outside by themselves, or being away from a parent. Then use the system outlined in this chapter to help your child confront those uncertainties and manage their own fears to gain independence.

- Talk openly about your child's fear and take them seriously.
- Discuss the end goal: freedom from the identified fear and a sense of independence.
- Work together to develop a plan. Start simple and, over the course of a month, slowly help your child take more control of the situation.
- Praise them when they meet a specific goal, like tucking themselves in at night or playing alone in their room for one hour.

Make sure to monitor your child's progress regularly and remember that this is a team effort. The goal is to help them to overcome and manage their fears. Never push the matter too hard or become angry and frustrated. If you see this happening, back away from the issue for a while, regroup, and readdress it again when you feel your child is ready.

Key Points

- Parents are responsible for the safety and security of their children. We are also responsible for teaching them to be independent and situationally aware. This requires us to have a firm understanding of the topics of awareness and personal safety.
- Understand the levels of awareness:

  1. Condition White: You're relaxed and unaware of what's going on. If you are ever attacked while in condition white, the chances of escape are diminished because your attacker will have caught you off guard.

  2. Condition Yellow: The preferable level of relaxed awareness. You appear to those around you to be entirely comfortable in your environment while paying close attention to the sights and sounds that surround you. You begin taking a mental inventory of your surroundings.

  3. Condition Orange: A possible threat has been identified, and you've narrowed your attention to that specific person or area. This is also the stage where you begin to put together spontaneous plans.

  4. Condition Red: This is where you find yourself right before you act on your plans. In condition red, the threat has materialized, and it's time to put those plans into action. This is also where the fight, flight, or freeze responses are triggered.

  5. Condition Black: Condition black is characterized by an excessively elevated heart rate (above 175 beats per minute) and a complete loss of cognitive ability. A person in condition black lacks the power to process the information being taken in effectively and becomes utterly useless in terms of response.

•Understand the reactionary gap and the OODA loop:

    1. Observe

    2. Orient

    3. Decide

    4. Act

• Comprehend the situation:

    1. Establish a baseline of behavior.

    2. Through observation, spot anomalies within the established baseline.

• Pay attention to intuition: Teach your child that if a situation feels wrong, get out of it.

• Spot the danger signs:

    1. Hidden hands

    2. Inexplicable presence

    3. Target glancing

    4. The sudden change of movement

    5. Inappropriate clothing

    6. Seeking a position of advantage

    7. Impeding your movement

    8. Unsolicited attempts at conversation

• Physiological signs of danger:

    1. Heavier than usual breathing

    2. Appearing tense

    3. Pupil dilation

    4. Excessive sweating

- Things to avoid:

    1. Teaching fear or using fear as a tool
    2. Focus lock on technology

- Help your child to manage their fear:

    1. Take your child's fear seriously.
    2. Work together.
    3. Give your child control.
    4. Don't use fear as a tool.

- Find a way out: Avoidance and escape are your child's two best options when it comes to personal safety.

2

How Children Learn New Tasks

"Tell me, and I forget. Teach me, and I remember.
Involve me, and I learn."
—BENJAMIN FRANKLIN

CHILDREN ARE LIKE LITTLE SPONGES. From the moment they take their first breath, they are learning. All five senses are fully engaged and taking in every possible detail about their new environment. You can see the amazement and curiosity on their faces as they try to make sense of it all. This process never stops. Children are continually finding new things that fascinate them. The endless stream of questions they can throw at us adults can sometimes be baffling and overwhelming. I'll admit it, I have no clue why God put a duckbill on a beaver ... Sometimes we have to prioritize the information we provide our children and help them to focus on what's most important at the moment. Crossing the street is not the time to wonder where rainbows come from; it's time to focus on the flow of traffic. When we start talking to our children about the world around them and what things are most important to their safety, we have to have a structured way of presenting this information. Given that we all learn in different ways, what's the best method for teaching these new, possibly life-saving concepts to our children?

Everyone, including your children, generally learns through three different mediums, visual, auditory, and tactile. Visual learners, who constitute almost half the population, learn best through sight. Auditory learners, who are less common, learn best by hearing; they remember the details of conversations and classroom lectures and may have strong language skills. Tactile learners learn best by doing and prefer more of a hands-on experience. Now let's break down each medium and consider what techniques work best for each individual learner.

Visual (Seeing):

- Provide visual aids such as pictures, charts, graphs, maps, flow-charts, diagrams, and timelines.
- Use multimedia presentations such as computers, videos, and PowerPoint.
- Use color to highlight important points in text.
- Illustrate ideas as a picture or brainstorming bubble before writing them down.
- Write a story and illustrate it.

Auditory (Hearing):

- Encourage discussions, debates, or teach-backs.
- Provide an opportunity for your child to recite the main points of a lesson or story.
- Allow them to read information out loud.
- Create musical jingles to aid memorization.
- Use analogies and storytelling to demonstrate your point.
- Encourage spoken answers to questions.

Tactile (Doing):

- Incorporate activities that allow for movement while learning (for example, hands-on use of a fire extinguisher).
- Ask them to take notes and encourage them to underline key points as you present your lesson.
- Use skits and role-plays to emphasize information.

The best way to ensure that your child is learning a new skill to their full potential is to incorporate all three methods of learning into your lessons. This is known as active learning, which is any learning endeavor in which the student participates or interacts with the learning process as opposed to passively taking in the information. The below illustration shows how active learning works best when it comes to actually retaining the information that's being presented.

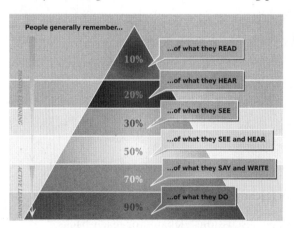

When I worked as an instructor for the Federal Air Marshal Service, we used the EDIP principle when it came to developing lesson plans and teaching our new candidates. EDIP stands for Explain, Demonstrate, Imitate, and Practice and incorporates all three methods of learning into the curriculum. We used this method to train thousands of federal air marshals, and I've found that these same principles work well when it comes to teaching children. Here's how the EDIP process breaks down:

31

- **Explain:** Give some background information on the topic and why it's important. Keep it short and simple so as not to confuse or distract anyone. Continue to explain as you move on to the next step. This is the auditory portion of the learning.
- **Demonstrate:** Demonstrate what you're teaching. Make sure that everyone can easily see and hear you. Avoid long explanations and pauses during the demonstration so that the learner can focus on observing the entire technique. This is the visual portion of the learning.
- **Imitate:** Get the learner to imitate the techniques you're teaching by mirroring you. That way, the learner can better understand its execution. Break things down into several sequences for easier learning if necessary. Give the required feedback and correction. This is where the "hands on" portion of learning a new task begins.
- **Practice:** Get the learner to practice the techniques. Note that it would not be reasonable to demand a high level of skill at this stage, as this would take more practice and time. Continue to give corrective and supporting feedback to encourage the learner to continue practicing. This is another tactical portion of the learning.

These principles worked well for us in the Federal Air Marshal Service, and can be easily adapted to teaching children about situational awareness. The trick is to find simple drills that work the fundamentals of awareness (nothing too complicated). Then modify those same exercises to be fun and instructive for children. Here's an example.

In my first book, *Spotting Danger Before It Spots You*, I outline a simple counting drill that can help adults to develop their situational awareness. These counting exercises are an effective way to maintain your focus when out in public. It takes discipline and conscious effort, but after a while, this technique becomes instinctive and greatly improves your chances of spotting a bad situation early. Here's how it goes:

- When you walk into a room, make it a habit to identify all of the exits.
- Count the number of people in your area, be it a restaurant, train, or parking lot.
- When counting, make sure to look at people's hands. The hands are what can hurt you.
- When walking down the street, periodically stop at a crosswalk or storefront and take a casual look behind you. Count the number of people who appear to be paying attention to what you do.
- When you're in a parking lot, count the number of cars with people sitting in them. How many of those cars are running?

This exercise requires close observation and concentration. To a potential attacker, this makes you look aware and focused, which makes you a less-appealing target. Now let's take the EDIP principles and adapt the same exercise to children:

- Explain to your child what you are going to be doing and why it's important. Counting can be fun, especially to younger children, so really emphasize the fact that you're about to do something exciting.
- Demonstrate using something simple like the number of exits, uniformed employees, or cars. Count them yourself and then tell your child the number you came up with. Ask them how quickly they think they could do the same.
- Allow them to imitate your actions by giving them something that they can count and keep track of, like the number of people in a checkout line at the store. Verify their numbers and encourage them to count other items as well. Keep track of their counting speed and praise them for counting accurately.
- Let them practice in different environments and with different things. Keep up the encouragement, and when you feel like the

game is becoming monotonous for the child, back off of it for a while and revisit it later. If you have multiple children or they're with friends, you can turn it into a contest. Nothing drives improvement like friendly competition.

When you're starting out, remember to use the processes of demonstration and imitation to help your child retain the methods you're teaching them. Some skills your child will learn are a little more complicated and require a specific sequence of actions. For these, you can break each task down into smaller steps. The idea is to teach the steps one at a time. When your child has learned the first step, then you teach the next, then the next, and so on. Move to the next step only when your child can do the previous one consistently and without your help. Eventually, they'll be able to perform the whole skill by themselves. We're going to get much deeper into games like these later on, and we'll see how this learning process can help to develop your child's memory, awareness, and critical thinking skills.

Now that you have a firm grasp on the EDIP principles, let's consider the best place to start when it comes to teaching children about situational awareness. As with any new skill, it's always best to start with the basics.

Kids in Action

T. J. Smith Stops a Kidnapping

One December in Wichita Falls, Texas, eleven-year-old T. J. Smith had just jumped off his scooter as his neighbor, Kim, and nine-year-old sister waited their turn. Kim was up next, and so she eagerly hopped on board and took off. As she made her way further down the sidewalk, a bearded man with a head full of messy curls appeared out of nowhere. Without uttering a word, he picked Kim up off the scooter and calmly strode away with her. "He cradled her like a baby and just walked down the street," says T. J. The composed way the man held Kim led T. J. to believe he might somehow be related to the little girl. But something wasn't right.

"I could see her face," T. J. said. "She was scared." Kim soon began to scream for help. She began kicking and punching, trying to get the man to let her go, but the man was unfazed. He continued walking down the street until he reached an alley and disappeared. T. J. admits that he was scared but says he never thought about the danger to himself. T. J.'s first impulse was to chase after the man who had taken his neighbor. "I wanted to help, but I couldn't do it myself," he said. So he ran to the house of a trusted neighbor. Brad Ware and his wife had been relaxing on the couch in their living room when T. J. burst through their front door. "Brad!" T. J. yelled. "A man just picked up a little girl and took her into the alley!" Then he took off again after the would-be kidnapper. "I ran back to where I saw him take her to see if they were still there," says T. J. Ware and his wife jumped into their car and followed T. J. down the street. T. J. ran to the end of the road and turned the corner. He had no idea what to expect or who might be waiting for him. But he needed to find Kim. If he lost her, T. J. feared, she might never be seen again. Once T. J. was in the alley, he spotted the strange man standing in front of an abandoned white house—its windows busted, doors boarded up, and yard overgrown. He was in the process of shoving little Kim through a window. Ware and his wife quickly pulled up to the scene. "Stay here," Ware told T. J. as he took off toward the house. With Ware now chasing him, the man let go of Kim and broke into a run. Ware caught up with him, and a struggle ensued. Ware kicked the man in the groin and gripped him in a bear hug. The man broke free and fled across the street. When he stumbled, Ware lunged and tackled him. T. J.'s little sister and a few other neighborhood kids alerted the police, who quickly arrived on the scene. Officers cuffed and arrested Raeshawn Perez, age twenty-six. He was charged with aggravated kidnapping.

There were several heroes that day, but Ware insists that it's T. J. who deserves most of the credit. "You know, he's the one who more or less saved the girl." That news came as no surprise to T. J.'s mother. "This is exactly his character," says Angie Hess Smith. "His first thought is not of himself. It's always of others." T. J.'s tenacity and quick thinking are shining examples of how situational awareness and intuition can save lives.[1]

---

1 "This 11-Year-Old Boy Saved His Friend from Being Kidnapped," https:// www.rd.com/true-stories/inspiring/stopping-a-kidnapper/

Exercise

Get used to using the EDIP method to teach your child new skills. Let them pick something that they'd like to learn, like finger painting, swinging a bat, or throwing a Frisbee. Then break that skill down using the methods outlined in chapter two.

- Explain the skill in simple terms that your child will understand.
- Demonstrate the skill to them.
- Allow them to imitate you as you both work on the skill together.
- Then allow them to practice the skill on their own. Remember that you need to be on hand to point out the proper corrections. You can always go back to the "demonstrate and imitate" phase if you feel like you need to.

As always, this is a team effort. Work together with your child to make sure they are learning the proper way to perform whatever skill they are pursuing. Be sure to praise them when they do well, and don't be afraid to back up and start over when it's warranted.

Key Points

- Active learning is any learning endeavor in which the student participates or interacts with the learning process, as opposed to passively taking in the information.
- People learn through three different mediums:

    1. Visual (seeing)
    2. Auditory (hearing)
    3. Tactile (doing)

- Two weeks after being presented with new information, we tend to remember:

    10% of what we read
    20% of what we hear
    30% of what we see
    50% of what we see and hear
    70% of what we say
    90% of what we do

- Children learn in many different ways. Use the EDIP method when teaching your child a new task:

    1. Explain: Give some background information on the topic and why it's important. Keep it short and simple so as not to confuse or distract anyone. Continue to explain as you carry on to the next step.
    2. Demonstrate: Demonstrate what you're teaching. Make sure that everyone can easily see and hear you. Avoid long explanations and pauses during the demonstration so that the learner can focus on observing the entire technique.
    3. Imitate: Get the learner to imitate the methods you're teaching by mirroring you. That way, the learner can better understand its execution. Break things down into several sequences for

easier learning if necessary. Give the feedback and correction needed.

4. Practice: Get the learner to practice the techniques. Note that it would not be reasonable to demand a high level of skill at this stage, as this would take more practice and time. Continue to give corrective and affirming feedback to encourage the learner to continue practicing.

• Use simple counting games when you're out in public to help get your child focused on their environment.

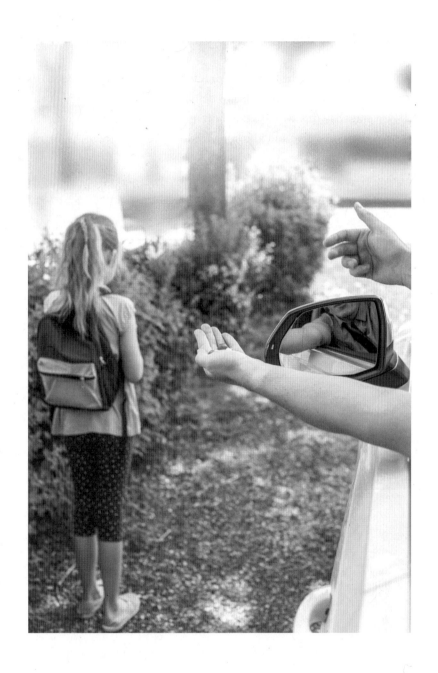

PHASE TWO——What Kids Need to Know

3

Teaching the Basics

"Success is neither magical nor mysterious. Success is the natural
consequence of consistently applying the basic fundamentals."
—JIM ROHN

I SPENT THREE YEARS working as a firearms instructor at the Federal Air
Marshal Services training center in Atlantic City, New Jersey. In that
time, I helped to train over five hundred of the world's finest shooters.
Some of the students we received had previous experience with a
handgun; others had never even held a firearm before they began their
training. Regardless of their skill level, the core curriculum remained
consistent. We always started out with the basics. Establishing a
proper stance and grip, then slow and steady draw strokes from con-
cealment. Then we followed up by reinforcing sight management, trigger control, and follow through. This progression was repetitive and
slow. If we saw something falling apart at this stage we would immediately stop to make the proper corrections and reset the process.
Once the fundamentals were understood and could be performed

properly and consistently, we started putting students on the clock. By slowly compressing the amount of time they had to complete a task, we would purposely "rush" the student to induce stress. When the fundamentals of marksmanship could be performed under these minimal levels of stress, we would find new and torturous ways to increase the stress levels until we were certain the student could execute the basics under any circumstances. Only then were they allowed to move on to the "advanced" portion of their firearms training. We did these things not to make life harder for our candidates but to instill in them one simple principle. At thirty thousand feet, pinpoint accuracy under extreme pressure was the only acceptable standard. The only way to ensure that standard was met was to continually stress the importance of the basics and to reinforce those fundamentals through training. Although much less stressful, teaching your child a new skill such as situational awareness is no different. You need to start with the basics, and then work your way slowly into the more complex aspects of situational awareness.

I generally recommend starting the conversation with your children about situational awareness between the pre-school ages of three and four. At this age, your children should be ready for a little more independence. By now, they're developing their organizational, social, and communication skills to the point that they can make themselves understood to others, even in times of crisis. Given the fact that your child will be spending more time separated from you, it's crucial that they can memorize and recite a few details about the adults in their lives. This will allow them to accurately relay that information to others in case of an emergency, so it's always a great place to start. Here are the five pieces of information that I recommend focusing on first:

1. **Parents' first and last names:** My wife used to work with small children as a nurse. Often, when she would ask a child the name of their parents, they would respond with "Mommy and Daddy." Make sure that as your children get older, you teach

them the right way to interact with the other adults they may come into contact with, especially those who may be there to help out in an emergency. Make sure your children know the proper first and last names of both parents and of anyone else in the family who may need to be contacted if something unexpected happens.

2. **Phone number:** This one was always a big one for my wife and me, especially once the kids were old enough to have their own phones. It's easy for them to put your number in their contacts list and forget it, but what if they need to dial you from a friend's phone or, God forbid, a hospital? When my kids were young, my wife would always sing the number to them in a catchy little jingle that she'd make up. Those can seriously get stuck in your head, and they'd often have several numbers memorized in a matter of hours. You can also have them practice dialing the number on a toy phone to help with the memorization.

3. **Home address:** Depending on the age of your child, this one may be harder to learn and can be broken down into smaller segments. Start by teaching your child the house number and street name. Once they can easily recite that, move on to the city, state, and zip code. When you're instructing your children about these more complicated pieces of information, be sure to help them whenever they get stuck and praise them often.

4. **Mom and Dad's place of work:** Some parents may not be able to take their phones into their place of employment. When I worked for the Bureau of Prisons, no phones were allowed inside the fence. If someone needed to get in touch with you, they would have to either know the number or be capable of looking it up. Kids may not have the number memorized, but they should be able to communicate the name of your workplace to someone else.

5. **A relative or trusted neighbor:** Let's face it. In the majority of cases, both parents are probably working and not always available during the day. Make sure your child knows at least the name and phone number of a close relative or trusted neighbor so that they can pass that information on to others in case of an emergency.

As your child is learning, make sure you have a back-up plan in the event they forget some of the details they've memorized. For instance, it's always a good idea to have this information written down and stored inside their backpack just in case. Make sure your child knows exactly where it's located, and don't keep it somewhere that's visible to others. Once your child is proficient at reciting everything, you can rest a little easier knowing that they can communicate effectively with other adults, or at least give them the necessary information they would need to contact a parent.

Now that your child has some basic identifying information memorized, it's time to start thinking about what specific skill sets they need to properly develop their situational awareness. Awareness in general can be broken down into three essential components: Identification, Comprehension, and Anticipation.

- Identification is the process of reading your environment based on the established baseline and identifying any behaviors that fall outside of that standard.
- Comprehension is the ability to quickly identify specific baseline anomalies and understand why that anomaly poses a risk to your security.
- Anticipation is the ability to visualize various possible outcomes based on the behaviors of the anomaly. Develop spontaneous plans of action based on the information you've gathered, and quickly choose the safest course of action.

This raises an important question: what specific skills will my child need to acquire and implement these essential components of situational awareness? The good news is that your child already does these things on a daily basis. Take, for instance, a child who just learned to ride their bike. That child is concentrating fully on one single task. As they peddle on their own, they scan their environment for anomalies. If the child identifies a problem, say an obstruction in their path, they comprehend the fact that if they strike the obstruction, they could be hurt. Now they start developing plans of action. They could strike the obstacle and risk injury, try to steer around the obstacle and risk losing control of the bike, or apply pressure to the breaks and steer the bike toward the soft grass on the edge of the path. The decision they make will be based on their ability to control their fear and focus on the end goal: personal safety. As a parent, there are certain things you can reinforce in your child that will help them to manage fear and keep them focused on making the best decision. Spatial awareness, problem-solving, and analytical thinking are the cognitive skills that heavily influence their ability to make the right choices. Let's take a closer look at each.

- Spatial awareness is your child's ability to know where they are in relation to other objects in their space and in what way those objects change in relation to how your child moves within that environment.
- Problem-solving is the process of finding solutions to complex issues. We do this by defining the problem; determining the cause; identifying, prioritizing, and selecting from among alternative solutions; and implementing the solution that works best.
- Analytical thinking is a critical component that gives one the ability to solve problems quickly and effectively. It involves a systematic step-by-step approach to thinking that allows you to break down complex problems into single, manageable components.

- Making a decision is the process of picking the best solution to a problem based on environmental conditions and taking action on that solution.

This may seem like complicated information for a child, but for now, we're not going to try to force-feed them this information and certainly not in these terms; we're going to package and present these skills in a way that children can both appreciate and enjoy ... through play.

Kids in Action

Braydon Smith Stops a Home Invasion

In Mebane, North Carolina, eleven-year-old Braydon Smith was on the phone with his mother one evening when suddenly a strange man came crawling through a ground floor window. The intruder was nineteen-year-old Jataveon Dashawn Hall. Once inside the home, Hall grabbed a pellet gun that was lying near the window and pointed it at Braydon. Hall then instructed Braydon to get into the closet. Braydon knew the gun was unloaded. As he slowly made his way toward the closet, he decided to make his move. "He went into the living room to grab my phone to make sure I didn't call 911 or anything. When I saw him try to put it in his pocket, I grabbed my machete off of my wall and went to hit him. I hit him in the back of the head," Braydon said. He had bought his machete with gift cards some time ago and usually used it to chop down trees.

But this time, he saw that it could be used as a self-defense weapon. Braydon credited his actions to a lesson his dad Christopher had taught him a few years earlier when burglars had broken into and ransacked their home. "If they come in the door, you let 'em have it," his dad had told him.

Braydon Smith said he was hesitant, but he wasn't scared. "It went by really fast. I knew I didn't have the time to think about what I was going to do. I just grabbed a weapon in the house and acted with it."

Local sheriff's deputies said the wounded intruder was later captured and taken into custody. When asked what advice he could give to others regarding such scary situations, Braydon responded, "Always have your kids prepared for anything."

Hall was later charged with breaking and entering, second-degree kidnapping, interfering with emergency communications, and assault on a child under twelve. The eleven-year-old had one more message for the intruder. "You shouldn't have done what you've done. You're better off to get a job than breaking into other people's houses."[1]

---

1 "11-Year-Old Boy Uses Machete to Stop Home Invasion," https://abc11. com/machete-11-year-old-attack-definition/5349431/.

Exercise

Use adjective flashcards like the one below to start teaching your child more descriptive words.

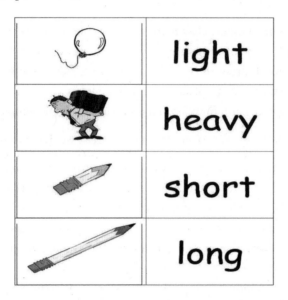

Once you feel like your child has a pretty good descriptive vocabulary, put it to the test.

When you're out in public, say at a park, pick out a person or an object and have them describe that person or object to you. Instead of saying something like "a man in a green jacket," have them be as specific as possible. "A tall, strong-looking man in a green jacket." The more they practice this, the more natural it will become. This skill will come in very handy if your child ever needs to describe you or a stranger who may have approached them.

Key Points

- Teach your children basic information that they can easily relate to another adult during emergencies:

  1. Parents' first and last name
  2. Parents' phone number
  3. Home address
  4. Mom and Dad's place of work
  5. The name and number of a relative or trusted neighbor

- Awareness can be broken down into three essential components:

  1. Identification is the process of reading your environment based on the established baseline and identifying any behaviors that fall outside of that standard.
  2. Comprehension is the ability to quickly identify specific baseline anomalies and understand why that anomaly poses a risk to your security.
  3. Anticipation is the ability to visualize various possible outcomes based on the behaviors of the anomaly. Develop spontaneous plans of action based on the information you've gathered, and quickly choose the safest course of action.

- There are three cognitive skills that heavily influence your child's ability to make the right choices in a given situation.

  1. Spatial awareness: Your child's ability to know where they are in relation to other objects in their space and in what way those objects change in relation to how your child moves within that environment.
  2. Problem-solving: The process of finding solutions to complex issues. We do this by defining the problem; determining the cause; identifying, prioritizing, and selecting from among alternative solutions; and implementing the solution that works best.

3. Analytical thinking: A critical component that gives one the ability to solve problems quickly and effectively. It involves a systematic step-by-step approach to thinking that allows you to break down complex problems into single and manageable components.

- Teaching your children about situational awareness and getting them dialed in to their surroundings will naturally build their curiosity and increase their attention span.

4

Game Night—Building a Foundation for Awareness

"For a small child, there is no division between playing and learning;
between the things he or she does 'just for fun' and things that are
'educational.' The child learns while living, and any part of living that
is enjoyable is also play."

—PENELOPE LEACH

CHILDREN ACQUIRE different intellectual skills as they meet certain developmental checkpoints. Many of these skills will be critical to the improvement of their situational awareness. You can help your child fully develop these abilities with fun, inexpensive, or even made-up games. Games spark your child's imagination and serve as a vehicle for education. They can help to improve memory, spatial awareness, comprehension, analytical thinking, problem-solving, and decision-making in a way that both the parent and the child can appreciate. More importantly, game night helps to reconnect the family. We are living in a time where individual and solitary activity is the norm. As electronic devices become more accessible, it's no longer unusual for children to have their own TVs, computers, and iPads, which mean that families seldom see the need to be in the same room together. As time goes on, it becomes harder and harder for us to connect with one another. Make it a point to schedule a game night at least two nights a week. For one or two hours, turn off the TV, set the phones aside, and just have fun. The life lessons your child learns will come naturally and they won't feel like work. According to family therapy and parent education specialist Marie Hartwell-Walker:

- Games teach important life skills. To win a game, one has to follow the directions, take turns, be patient, and stay friendly with the others around the table. Many games require us to strategize, to read others' nonverbal cues, and to learn from our own errors. Regular game nights give kids practice in these essential skills and provide immediate feedback about what works and what doesn't.
- Games teach good sportsmanship. Kids aren't born good sports. They tend to gloat when they win and whine when they lose. Most kids try cheating at least once. Games provide opportunities for kids to learn that honest winning feels better and makes better relationships than cheating. They provide a forum for teaching children how to be gracious winners and good losers.
- Playing together fosters family communication. As kids get older, the in-between times become the times when the most important conversations occur. Kids are more likely to share their thoughts and feelings when they are doing something else. The times between turns, between hands of cards, and between games are fertile ground for casual sharing of sometimes not-so-casual information.

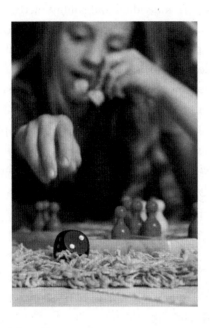

Family game nights are a great way to create positive memories. Families that can have fun together on a regular basis create an emotional "bank" of good memories and positive feelings that can be drawn on when things go bad or when family members find themselves apart. Those trying times are when children will be able to tap into the skills they've learned through play and apply them to broader concepts of situational awareness and personal safety, which we'll learn later on.

In this chapter, we'll look at several popular family games and see how each one helps develop various components of situational awareness. Later on you'll see how each component ties into a specific aspect of situational awareness. It's crucial that you recognize these individual skills so you can emphasize them during game night. Here are a few games my wife and I used to play with our children to help get you started.

- *Memory*: I'm sure a lot of you remember this game from your childhood. It's a simple card game where cards displaying various objects are laid out in a grid pattern. Each card has a match somewhere in the grid. Players take turns flipping over two cards. If they match, that player keeps the cards. If they don't match, they're returned to their original position, and the next player gets a turn. Once the grid is depleted, the player with the most matches wins. I used to love playing this game with the kids. It's best suited for children ages three to twelve and is a great way to start developing their memory as well as their concentration. Memory plays a big role in situational awareness training, especially when it comes to relaying specific events to others. For instance, if a stranger approached your child, you would want them to be able to accurately relay detailed information about that person. What were they wearing? What color was their hair? Were they short or tall? You get the picture. All of this information is going to come from the child's memory, so you want them to start developing those skillsets as early as possible.

- **I Spy**: I Spy is a fun game that can be played just about anywhere. At home, on a road trip, in a restaurant—the possibilities are endless. The game usually goes like this. The parent will say, "I spy with my little eye" and then give the child a descriptor of whatever it is they want them to identify. For instance, if the parent is looking at a tree, they would maybe start with the word green, and then move on to the word tall, and so on until the child identifies the correct object. Then it's the child's turn to pick an object for you to guess. This game is a great way to develop the child's powers of observation as well as their ability to be descriptive. More importantly, it keeps their head up and their minds alert to their surroundings, which is a habit you want them to maintain as they get older.

- **What's Missing:** This one is a variation on a KIM's game, or keep-in-memory game. A variety of random items are laid out on a table or a tray. Allow your child to study the items for as long as they'd like. Then have them occupy themselves for a little while doing something else. The amount of time you give your child to study the items and the time they take away can be varied as they get better at the game. After a set period, have them return to the items; however, this time make sure that you've taken something away from the original display. Ask your child, "What's missing?" and see if they can identify the correct item. This game is great for developing memory, but it's also a fantastic way for them to begin thinking in terms of "What's wrong with this picture?" which will greatly increase their ability to spot baseline anomalies when they get to that stage of their training.

- **Spot the Good Guy:** Fred Rogers once said, "When I was a boy, and I would see scary things in the news, my mother would say to me, 'Look for the helpers. You will always find people who are helping.'" Find the Good Guy is a game my wife made up. When she was out with the children, she would always have them identify the people around them who were considered the "good guys" and could be trusted to help in an emergency. She would then have them explain why they identified that person. These good guys naturally consisted of police officers, paramedics, firefighters, and nurses, but she also taught them to look more closely at those who weren't as easily recognizable. Store employees and mothers or fathers with children of their own were always plentiful and easy to spot. Have your child keep count of the good guys they identify and the location where they saw them. (We will consider a more detailed version of this game in chapter 6.)

- **Drive Us Home:** This one is simple. When you have your children out in the car, allow them to give you directions back home. Ask them questions along the way. Do we turn here? Do we turn left or right? Do you know how many stoplights we'll hit between here and home? The older the child, the more complicated the questions can be. This exercise is fantastic for building spatial awareness. As your child becomes better at the game, you can mix it up by taking different routes and passing different landmarks like police stations, hospitals, and firehouses. You can also use this game when you're out walking to better familiarize your child with your neighborhood, shopping mall, or local park.

- *Clue*: A popular board game for children between the ages of eight and twelve, the object of the game is to solve a murder. Who did it? With what weapon? In which room? As you make suggestions about the murder suspect, weapon, and location, you will eliminate possibilities and get closer to the truth. This is a fantastic game for families to play together and helps to build your child's critical thinking skills and deductive reasoning. These skills are critical when it comes to the planning stages of situational awareness.

- **Chess:** I love chess. I'm no expert, but I love and appreciate the skills that chess teaches. They're skills that can be applied to daily life on almost every level, and they're important skills to have when it comes to building situational awareness. Chess is simple enough to play once you learn all the moves, but the level of complexity required to win is immense. I'll avoid talking about rules and moves and focus on the important skills that can be learned on the board. Chess improves memory and pattern recognition. It develops strategic thinking, critical thinking, planning, and foresight. Your child's ability to look at a real-life situation, identify the players, spot patterns, and develop plans is critical to their survival. I highly recommend teaching your child how to play chess (or learning it yourself) and as they progress, emphasize the importance of each of these skills and how they translate to situational awareness.

- **Role-Playing:** This one was always a favorite of my wife's. Role-playing is a fantastic way to help build awareness because it requires visualization. As the old saying goes, "your body will not go where your mind hasn't been." Visualization techniques have been proven to improve performance in almost every way. In my first book, I relay the story of James Nesmeth. A POW during the Vietnam War, Mr. Nesmeth loved to golf. As he was locked away in his cell, he visualized every detail of the game he loved—the setup, adjusting for the wind, the swing, and the flight of the ball. He did this every day of his incarceration. When he was finally released and returned home, the first thing he wanted to do was play a game of golf. Despite not touching a club for seven years, Nesmeth golfed the best game of his life that day, and he attributed the whole thing to his routine of visualization. Role-playing not only requires visualization. It requires you to react to things physically. My wife would often approach my children as if she was a drug dealer and ask them, "Hey kid, you want to get high?" To which my children knew to shout, "NO! Get away from me!" The very thought of my sweet little wife trying to sell drugs to children is absurd in the extreme, but the lesson she was teaching was invaluable. She understood that by practicing that reaction now, it would be easier for them to have the same reaction if they were approached by a stranger later on. We used these same principles in the Federal Air Marshal Service when we would practice hijacking scenarios on the aircraft simulators. Nothing fires the mind quicker than being attacked by a determined man with an electronic shock knife whose main objective is to incapacitate you and gain access to the cockpit. This type of role-playing is taken to the extreme, but it's a necessary exercise if you expect to develop the proper reactions to violence.

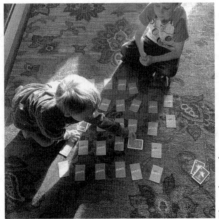

Photo by author

Game night with my nephews.

Let's face it: some adults are going to be apprehensive about talking to their child about situational awareness because they're afraid that it will lead to subjects that they're just not ready to talk about yet, and that's okay. Just break out the games and start working on the skills your child will need down the road when you are ready to broach the issues of danger and predatorial violence. All of these games, and many like them, are wonderful ways to get your child used to observing details, asking specific questions, and thinking critically about their environment. These are also skills that are critical to the process of becoming situationally aware. I only listed a few of the games we used to play as a family and you can add to this list as much as you like. You are only limited by your imagination; just remember what skills you want to emphasize when you're choosing a game and how each of those skills helps to reinforce the necessary elements of situational awareness.

As a side note, make sure you are fully involved when playing these games. Turn off the television, put away the cell phones, and have your child do the same. Your kids have to realize that it's okay to disconnect from technology once in a while. In the following chapters, as we start to get more into the meat and potatoes of building situational awareness for children, the ability to get your head up and focus solely on your surroundings will be an invaluable lifesaving skill. It's crucial your children understand that. Now let's take a look at the abilities your child has built through play and apply those to real-world situational awareness.

Kids in Action

Eyas Tran Saves His Neighbor

One Wednesday afternoon, in Hampton, New Hampshire, Eyas Tran was walking with his parents when he noticed a newspaper on his neighbor's doorstep. Eyas enjoyed bringing the newspaper to their elderly neighbor, Peggy. "We consider her family," said Eyas's mom. When Eyas got to her door, though, he noticed that a few other papers had piled up. "There was one, two, three newspapers," Eyas said. He quickly alerted his parents, who knew something must be wrong when Peggy didn't answer the door or her phone. Once they realized that her car was still parked in the garage, they decided to call the police. When officers arrived, they found Peggy in her basement. She had somehow locked herself down there for three days. Deputy Police Chief David Hobbs said, "It was just one of those freak accidents where the door closed behind her, and she was stuck downstairs." She was taken to the hospital but was soon released. Police say if it weren't for little Eyas, who knows how long his favorite neighbor may have been down there? "We truly thank this young boy for his actions in alerting his mother," said Deputy Chief Hobbs. "We just want to say to everybody else, be more like Eyas. Check on your neighbors. Look after each other."[2]

---

2 "Three-Year-Old NH Boy Helps Save Elderly Neighbor Trapped in Basement for Days," https://boston.cbslocal.com/2020/05/07/ hampton-new-hampshire-police-woman-in-basement/.

Exercise

KIM's Game

KIM's games, which I refer to in my first book, *Spotting Danger Before It Spots You*, are commonly used in military and law enforcement sniper training to increase observational skills. What most people don't know is that the game originally derived from the Rudyard Kipling novel, *Kim*. In the novel, the game is called both "The Play of the Jewels" and "The Jewel Game." The protagonist, Kim, spends a month at the home of his mentor, Mr. Lurgan, who as a cover runs a jewel shop but in truth is a British spy working against the Russians. Lurgan brings out a copper tray, tosses a handful of jewels onto it, and then instructs Kim, " Look on them as long as thou wilt, stranger. Count and, if need be, handle. One look is enough for me. When thou hast counted and handled and art sure that thou canst remember them all, I cover them with this paper, and thou must tell over the tally ..." They play the game many times, sometimes with jewels, sometimes with odd objects, and sometimes with photographs of people. It is considered a vital part of Kim's training in observation.

In basic training for the Federal Air Marshal Service, candidates are given several random objects to memorize in a short period and then asked about what they saw later in the day. As the training progresses, the number of objects increases, as does the amount of time between observation and questioning. This helps to build the candidate's level of awareness, attention to detail, and memory. It's also a fun game you can play with your children to help them hone those same skills.

Lay several random items out on a tray; start simple with only three or four things, and as your child progresses, keep adding to the number. Have them memorize as much of what they see as possible, taking in as much detail as they can. Then have them occupy themselves with something else for a while so that they forget about the items on the tray. After a while, call them back and ask them questions about what they saw. Take note of how much they remember. As they get better at the game, you can add more and more items, and increase the amount of time they are away from the tray. KIM's games are a great way to improve memory and hone observational skills. They're easy to set up yourself or you can find them on the Internet. And the more you practice them, the better you'll get. You can also apply this concept to your child's environment.

The next time you're in the grocery store, have your child pay attention to the cashier. Once you're back in the car, start asking them questions. What color was the cashier's hair? Were they wearing glasses? Did you happen to see a name on their nametag? When presented as a game and associated with something fun, children become more attentive to their environment and are much more willing to participate.

Key Points

Children learn best when they're having fun. Basic games are a great way to teach necessary situational awareness skills such as:

- Spatial awareness
- Problem-solving skills
- Analytical thinking
- Decision-making

Games also teach:

- Important life skills. These include how to follow directions, take turns, be patient, and stay friendly with the others around the table.
- Good sportsmanship. Games provide opportunities for kids to learn that honest winning feels better and makes better relationships than cheating.
- Family communication. Kids are more likely to share their thoughts and feelings when they are doing something else.

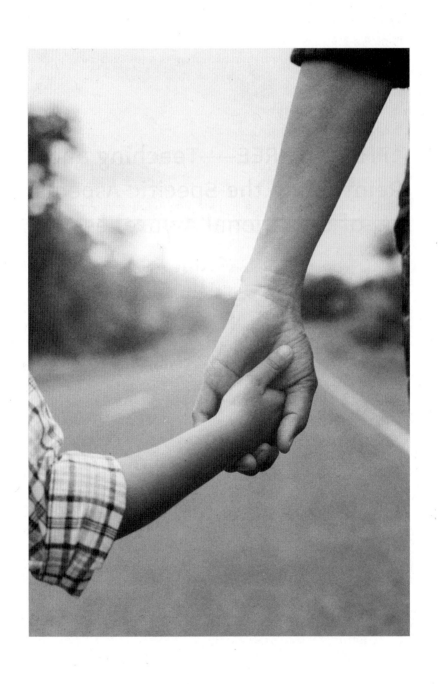

PHASE THREE—Teaching and Reinforcing the Specific Aspects of Situational Awareness

5

Situational Awareness for Children

"An observant child should be put in the way of things worth
observing."
—CHARLOTTE MASON

UP TO THIS POINT, you should be familiar with the basic elements of
situational awareness, the skill sets that are required to maintain that
awareness, and how these skills are applied to children through play.
We've also covered how our children can learn new skills through the
EDIP principle. Now it's time to start developing a plan to pass that
information on to your child in a way that sparks their interest without inducing unreasonable fear. I say unreasonable because I feel that
a little apprehension is a good thing. It fosters a natural sense of cau-
tion without triggering the anxiety caused by irrational phobias. A
little fear can be managed through concentration and observation,
paired with confidence in your own ability. The skills that your child
has developed through gameplay can now be directed toward building
that confidence. As we move through the following sections, your

child will start to understand how the abilities they've developed through play can now be applied to their everyday lives. As they progress through this journey to situational awareness, you'll see that the recognition of these new skills will promote a steady increase in their self-reliance and a willingness to learn more. But it's important to remember that our children view the concept of danger in a different light than we do.

Situational awareness and preparedness are a little unique for children. They don't have the natural defenses that we adults do. Adults can hit the gym or the dojo to harden themselves up. We can legally arm ourselves, and we have a better understanding of how the world works in general. Children, on the other hand, are small and not very intimidating. They haven't developed that natural skepticism that most adults have about other people in general. Children's security comes from their ability to observe their surroundings, identify threatening situations, and communicate those threats to the adults around them. That's their best defense against danger, and it's important that we as adults give them the tools they need to properly develop those skills. That means that we adults owe it to our children to educate ourselves on the dangers out there.

Rory Miller, author of *Meditations on Violence*, points out that there are two types of predators among us: resource predators and process predators. A resource predator is looking for something valuable, like money, jewelry, or an unguarded laptop. They've decided they need some physical item and they're going to find someone to take it from. Predators in this category include your basic mugger, pickpocket, or burglar. In some cases, if a resource predator confronts you and you just give them the thing they want, they go away. The process predator, on the other hand, is much different. The process predator isn't interested in your watch or briefcase; they get off on the act of violence itself. This category of predator includes the likes of rapists and murderers. When you look at how this applies to children, the resource predator may view your child as a source of income, be it through kidnapping for ransom or selling the child into human trafficking. Process predators, on the other hand, do not change. They're still in it for the sheer violence and the feeling it gives them. It's hard to come to grips with the fact that another human being could be so cruel and callous toward a child, but the truth is that thousands of children are kidnapped, murdered, sexually abused, or sold into human trafficking every year. No decent human being wants to imagine their child suffering such a fate; that's why it's so important that we be proactive and start teaching our children the core objectives of situational awareness at an early age. These core objectives include:

1. Understanding normal environmental behaviors.
2. Spotting abnormal environmental behaviors.
3. Planning a means of avoidance or escape should a dangerous situation present itself.
4. Taking action on those plans.

Now we'll break down each of these objectives and look specifically at how they can be applied to children.

5.1 Understanding Normal Behaviors

I explained earlier how the baselines of behavior are established. Now it's time to start letting your child's cognitive skills take the wheel as we guide them through this process. It all starts before you ever leave the house. It's easy to sit down with your child and have a conversation about the places they will go. Let's say, for instance, that you plan on taking your child to the park. Before you leave the house, start asking them questions about what they think they'll see there. "Will there be other children in the park?" "Will the other people there be happy or sad?" "How do you think everyone will be dressed?" Questions like this will start firing the process of visualization and allow your child to draw some general conclusions about baseline behaviors before you ever get there. If your child has been there before, they should have a pretty good idea of what to expect. By talking about their expectations beforehand, they'll be better able to speak with you about the things they feel are out of place or make them feel uncomfortable.

When you get to your destination, the first thing you should do is have your child express their general feeling about the place based on what they expected from the baseline. Here's a good way to practice that. The next time you walk into an area, be it a park, a restaurant, or shopping mall, give your child a few minutes to acclimate to their new surroundings, and then ask them this simple question: "How does this place make you feel?" Depending on their age, you may get a range of answers. "Happy." "Sad." "Good." "Bad." "I don't feel like anything." What's important is that you follow up, asking questions like, "What about this place makes you feel that way?" or "If you feel frightened, why?" Allow your child to express their feelings, but always try to ask a few probing questions to pinpoint the source of their concerns. When you do, have your child be as descriptive as possible about anything that may be making them apprehensive. If the feeling they get is good, have them be specific about what it is that makes them feel that way. Their answers regarding good feelings should reflect normal baseline behaviors.

Once the baseline is established, start diving into some of the games we talked about earlier. Spot the Good Guy is always a good place to start. Have your child identify as many helpers as they can as you move through your environment, and be sure to have them articulate why they chose the people they did. Were they in uniform? Were they wearing a nametag? Did they have children? *Memory* is also an excellent game to play in this circumstance. You could have them memorize the number of good guys they spotted and where they were located. Have them point to the direction of the exits or to where your car is parked. The point is to keep them fully engaged with their surroundings. As they play these little games, what they're actually doing is a detailed scan. They may not know it at the time, but their constant interaction with their surroundings has them open and alert to any changes within that environment. This brings us to the next objective of situational awareness, spotting abnormal behavior.

5.2 Spotting Abnormal Behaviors

Now that the baseline is established and you have your child fully engaged with their surroundings, they have to start identifying things that may be out of place or make them feel uncomfortable. Anytime they see or feel anything that makes them apprehensive or afraid, they must know their first move should be to come to you with the problem. If for some reason you aren't nearby, they should alert one of the preselected good guys to the issue. In my first book, *Spotting Danger Before It Spots You*, I tell the story of Julianne Moore. Julianne was a typical eleven-year-old girl who lived with her parents and younger brother Hayden in the suburbs just outside of Cleveland, Ohio. In the spring of 2019, Julianne and her brother were playing in the front yard near the street while her parents worked in the back. That's when a strange man approached the two children and tried to engage them in conversation. In subsequent interviews with the media, Julianne said, "He started to talk to us, but we really couldn't figure out what he was saying. It was like gibberish, so we really didn't think much of it." Julianne knew most of the adults in her neighborhood, and something about this man didn't feel right. As the man walked away, Julianne kept a close eye on him. She noticed that he hesitated and circled back toward them, another behavior that gave her a bad feeling. She quickly moved closer to her brother as the stranger lunged for Hayden and tried to pull him away by his arm. Julianne said, "When he tried to grab my brother, I knew, like this was serious. I just grabbed my brother and went into the backyard because there was no time to panic. You just have to go with it." The children's father, Joshua Moore, told reporters, "My daughter came running back there with my son, dragging him by the arm and said, 'A man tried to abduct Hayden!'" At that point, Joshua ran to the front of the house and confronted the stranger, who continued walking away. He then called the police. Young Julianne had remained calm and observant during the incident and gave the police a detailed description of the stranger, including what he looked like, what he was wearing, and which direction he was headed. Using her report, police located the man nearby, placed him under arrest, and charged.him with attempted abduction. Looking back on the incident, Julianne said she was still rattled by what happened but was grateful that her parents had taught her to remain calm when faced with an emergency and to always to keep an eye on her little brother. Julianne's ability to react to her intuition, remember as much detail about the stranger as possible, and quickly alert her parents was instrumental in saving her brother and resolving the situation. This scenario is a perfect example of how everything can be fine one second and turn horribly wrong the next. That's why it's crucial to make sure your children are tuned in to their surroundings. Use the games we've discussed to help them make a habit of awareness. That way, when a baseline anomaly does present itself, they're not caught off guard and can react quickly to the change.

5.3 Creating a Plan

Young Julianne clearly had a plan: fight to save her brother and alert her parents as soon as possible—pretty straightforward. Some of her actions were completely subconscious. Despite her obvious fear, she was aware enough to take in a full description of the man and note what direction he was headed. This gave the police the information they needed to track the man down and make an arrest. Planning doesn't have to be overly complicated. When it comes to training your children in situational awareness, simplicity is always the best option.

Now let's give some thought to situations where planning is a critical element in safety and security. Although the dangers of kidnapping and predatorial violence are very real, it's much more likely that children will find themselves in situations around their own homes that require a preplanned response. Natural disasters and medical emergencies occur without warning and can cause a significant amount of fear and confusion in a young child. We adults must take the time to explain what constitutes an actual emergency and work with our children to create step-by-step plans for how to react in those situations.

Dr. Sanam Hafeez is a New York-based child psychologist who developed a specific program that outlines what kids can do in case of a crisis. Dr. Hafeez says the first step is teaching your young one to recognize what can actually be considered an emergency. "Your child could literally be in an emergency and not realize it," she says. This knowledge comes directly from her personal experience. "When I was eight years old, my house caught fire. And I was in my room reading a book. I had no idea what was happening," she says. "My sister came and got me, and I still didn't quite understand— no one had ever really spoken to us about an emergency, and I said to my sister, 'Oh, I think I should get my bike.' I was a bright kid, and my parents were very hands-on, but it just goes to show you kids don't understand the devastation something like a fire can cause."

Before you can get serious about developing plans of action, you have to teach your child that not everything is an emergency. You can't find your fairy wings ... not an emergency. Optimus Prime is missing his head ... not an emergency. You come home from school, and the door is broken and standing open—that's an emergency! Dr. Hafeez recommends explaining it like this: "An emergency is something very serious or very dangerous, like if Mommy or Daddy is hurt and can't get to the phone, or you're alone, and no one can come to you for help, or someone's trying to break in the door, or there are bad people in the house," she says. "Go ahead and give them a range of scenarios, but remember they're designed to teach, not terrify."

When you develop these emergency scenarios for your children, make sure you give them easy-to-follow instructions, and if at all possible, have them act out their responses. This will help them to "break the freeze" and take action during an emergency, even though they may be scared. Let's take a look at a couple of common examples.

Scenario 1

Question: You're outside playing, and your brother falls off his bike. He's crying and says that his arm hurts really bad, and you see that it's bleeding a little. What should you do?

Answer: Ask if he's okay; make sure he is in a safe place away from traffic. Get him into the house if he can walk. If not, get an adult.

Scenario 2

Question: Mommy falls in the living room and hits her head. She is bleeding. When you ask if she's okay, she doesn't answer. What should you do?

Answer: If no other adults are in the house, get to the phone and call 911. Tell them my name and that there is an emergency. Tell them what's happening and give them our address. Stay on the phone if they ask me to, and open the door when help arrives.

Scenario 3

Question: You come home from school and notice that the front door is standing open. The lock looks like it has been broken. You can see inside and notice that the furniture is turned over and there appears to be broken glass on the floor. What should you do?

Answer: Go to a trusted neighbor's home and tell them what has happened. Ask to call 911. (If your child is younger, it may be a good idea to have them ask the neighbor to call 911 for them. If your child has a cellphone, they can call 911 immediately.) Tell the dispatcher what has happened and that someone I do not know may be in the house. Give them my name and address. Let them know that I am across the street at the neighbor's house and stay there until the police arrive.

Those are just a few examples of emergencies that may require a response from your child, but everyone is different. When you begin this type of training, it's imperative that you understand how much your child can handle. Kids in every age group will respond differently to stress. Start with simple, less-frightening scenarios. Once your child is comfortable with what's expected of them, add a few contingencies to make them a little more complex. Pay close attention to your child's responses. Allow them to think freely about how they should react, but don't let them stray too far from the plan. Make sure they understand the main objective: to keep themselves and their family safe and free from danger.

On December 6th, 2019, a four-year-old girl name Isla Glaser saved her mother's life by quickly responding to a medical emergency and calling 911. She was at her home in Franklin Township, New Jersey, with her mom, Haley Glaser, and three younger siblings, when Haley had a medical episode and collapsed. Little Isla found her mother's cell phone and calmly called 911. "My mommy falled down, and she can't talk," Isla told the 911 dispatcher. She then answered several questions and gave the dispatcher her address before letting them know that her father was at work and she was home with her three younger siblings. Not only did Isla keep her siblings calm, she also controlled her family's large dogs when emergency responders came to the door. On the recorded call, you can hear Isla yell: "Puppies get out of the way! Puppies get out of the way!" Once inside the home, medics rushed unconscious Haley to the hospital where she spent several days due to a bacterial infection. "I know adults that cannot handle that kind of incident with that much bravery, poise, and distinction," Lt. Philip Rizzo of the Franklin Township Police Department said at a news conference. "For that, this young lady needs to be commended."

Little Isla Glaser was hailed a hero by her community, and this is just one example of many where children under the age of six have leapt into action to save a loved one. We all like to think that our children would act similarly, but the truth of the matter is that these types of reactions very seldom "just happen." They have to be discussed, and practiced regularly. Take the time to teach your kids things like the location of fire extinguishers, first aid kits, and medical equipment. If you really want to be a superstar, make arrangements to take them to the local firehouse. There they can meet actual firefighting men and women, ask questions, and maybe sit in a fire truck. Some firehouses are even equipped with bedroom simulators where your children can learn how to escape to safety in the event of a house fire. These live rehearsals, whether practiced at home, at school, or in a firehouse, help to build muscle memory so your child can act decisively and with confidence in the event of an actual emergency.

The structured scenarios I outlined earlier are a great way to get your child thinking about safety and security. This safety mindset, paired with the skills they've picked up through games, can significantly improve their ability to respond to emergencies they haven't necessarily prepared for. Just like young Julianne and Isla, your child can not only develop the ability to spot dangerous situations before they materialize, they can immediately anticipate outcomes and develop plans to ensure their safety and the safety of others. That alone is a pretty impressive set of skills, but once the threat is present, a whole new set of circumstances reveal themselves. Anytime a person is faced with an unexpected emergency, it can trigger the stress responses of fight, flight, or freeze. These stress responses can be incredibly intense, especially with children, so it's crucial that we teach them how to confront their fears and act on their plans.

5.4 Taking Action

Before we can effectively discuss your child's ability to act in an emergency, it's important that you have an understanding of what causes the fight, flight, or freeze response in both adults and children. The human nervous system is broken into two parts: the sympathetic nervous system (SNS) and the parasympathetic nervous system (PNS). The SNS is what mobilizes and directs the body's energy resources and prepares you for action. It also triggers your adrenal glands to flood your body with adrenaline. When this happens, certain things occur physically that you'll need to be aware of beforehand. Your heart rate and breathing will speed up so blood and oxygen can be rushed to the muscles to prep them for a fight. Your pupils will dilate, and you could lose your peripheral vision, which causes you to experience "tunnel vision." You could also experience what's known as auditory exclusion, which is to say that under severe stress, the processing of auditory inputs may become muted, or even completely shut down. Another harmful physical side effect is the deterioration of fine motor skills. You experience a tingling in your hands and feet caused by blood vessels constricting, forcing blood away from your extremities and causing it to pool around your internal organs to protect them from damage. This can cause your fingers, arms, and legs to feel week and clumsy. The SNS is also what triggers your fight, flight, or freeze responses. The option you pick isn't really up to you, at least not to your rational thinking self. When the SNS is triggered, we tend to go into what I call the "big dumb animal mode." We cease to think rationally, and the big dumb animal inside of us takes over. But like any animal, the big dumb one inside of us can be trained to give the right response. All of these responses triggered by the SNS are natural, and they occur with everyone, including your child. The trick is to teach them how to break the freeze response and act. Let's now take a look at a few options you have when teaching children to take action.

The scenarios we discussed earlier are a great way to give your child a structured plan of action for a given situation. The more scenarios you can come up with and work through with your child, the better prepared they'll be. But what happens when something unexpected pops up? What happens when your child is faced with an unforeseen, stress-inducing event? How will they react? The best way to begin this discussion with your child is to be open and honest about what they can expect from themselves. They may not be at the age where they fully understand the difference between the PNS and SNS, but they might be fully capable of expressing their fears. Earlier in chapter 1, we discussed ways to help your child manage those fears, but what's the best way to get them to take action in the face of uncertainty? The answer to that question is by building confidence. As a firearms instructor for the Federal Air Marshal Service, I've always found that confidence comes from competence. Once a skill has been mastered and can be demonstrated under stress, the student becomes confident in their ability to perform the task under any conditions. This leads to a change in the way they feel, the way they think, and the way they act. Your child is no different. Their ability to master and demonstrate skills is what gives them confidence, and that's the one thing they need to move forward.

Believe it or not, your child is already well on the way to being a confident, self-sufficient individual. Just take a look at what we've covered so far. They've memorized all of the necessary information they need to communicate effectively with adults during a crisis. On game night, your child has built a foundation for awareness and improved their memory, cognitive processing, critical thinking skills, and deductive reasoning. They've learned to understand normal behaviors and spot baseline anomalies. They've been given plans of action for how to react to specific emergencies and demonstrated through practice the full range of their capabilities. As a parent, you have to stay engaged and make sure your child understands just how vital these skills are. Impress upon them how proud you are that they've come this far and how certain you are that they can act appropriately in an emergency. This alone will help to build their confidence and give them the courage they need to act on their own. In the end, this is what we want for our children: to be able to monitor their surroundings and act decisively and independently when an emergency arises. The skill sets are there. Now we need to make sure your child understands their full range of options and under what circumstances each option is warranted.

Kids in Action

Dylan Paul Saves His Teacher

Dylan Paul is a fifth-grade student. One day while in his computer class, he noticed something was wrong with his teacher, Karen Renko. Karen had been eating a muffin when suddenly she wasn't able to breathe. Thankfully, young Dylan, who had just watched a YouTube video on performing chest thrusts, came to the rescue. "All of a sudden, she starts doing the universal choking sign, which I see," Dylan said. "I get out of my chair, and I ask her if she is choking." "What I did was I propped right up at the sternum, and then I would pull back," Dylan explained. "And then somebody else, the other kids in my class, went to go get teachers to help, but when they got there … she had already stopped choking." Dylan, whose efforts dislodged the obstruction, felt like he was paying his teacher back with his good deed. "I am very thankful for what she has done for me," he said. "So, I think it kind of made it even." Karen was very grateful that Dylan was nearby and so willing to act. "I am so thankful to have had Dylan in the room at the time," she said. "His presence of mind and willingness to step up and help show that he is wise beyond his years. Dylan is a real live hero."[3]

---

3 "5th-Grader Awarded Certificate for Saving Teacher," https://www.wnem.com/news/th-grader-awarded-certificate-by-sheriff-for-saving-teacher/article_8625579c-70f0-11e9-b94a-b708759b481d.html.

Exercise

Reading the Room

The next time you're out in public, teach your child to "read the room." It's a very simple exercise that will help your child to spot potentially dangerous situations and improve their awareness. Here's how it works.

The next time you drop your child off at school or daycare, take some time before you leave to ask them a few simple questions:

- How do you think everyone is feeling here today?
- Do you see anyone who looks happy?
- Do you see anyone who looks like they may be sad or afraid?
- What kind of mood do you think your teacher is in based on how she's acting right now?

Have them be as descriptive as possible and be specific about why they feel the way they do about those they identify. Questions like these will get your child used to taking a few moments to read the mood of a room or a situation before they fully commit themselves to it. The reason you want to do this in an environment they're familiar with is because they'll already have a pretty good idea of the baseline of behavior. They know how people generally act in that environment so they can spot anomalies much quicker.

Key Points

• The basics of awareness for children:

1. Help your child to understand and identify normal behaviors within their environment.
2. Point out the things that concern you and have them point out the things that they feel are abnormal behaviors.
3. Use simple games and visualization techniques to help your child develop a plan of action.
4. Teach your child that not every situation is dangerous. Make sure they understand what is and what isn't an emergency.

6

Give Your Children Options

"You have brains in your head. You have feet in your shoes. You can steer
yourself any direction you choose. You're on your own. And you know
what you know. And YOU are the one who'll decide where to go …"

—DR. SEUSS

IT'S BEEN SAID that having only one option is no option at all. I'm a
firm believer in that. I like to have options, and being placed in a situation where there's only one way out makes me apprehensive. Earlier,
I spoke about playing counting games with your children when you're
out in public. Counting the number of exits, windows, employees,
police officers—we do this to make the habit of paying attention fun
for our children, but it also serves another purpose. When it comes to
the planning stages of reacting to potential danger, all of this information helps your child to make a decision and gives them options. We
want our kids to understand that there is always more than one way
to solve a problem. By allowing them to think through their situation

and identify as many solutions as possible, we're giving them the tools they need to act in the face of danger as opposed to freezing.

There's something known as Hick's Law that describes the time it takes a person to make a decision as a result of the possible choices he or she has. Increasing the number of options also increases the time it takes to make a decision. This concept was first put forward by British psychologist William Edmond Hick and is widely taught in law enforcement circles. But there's a common misconception regarding Hick's Law that I think needs a little clarification. Most people believe that by adding multiple solutions to a problem they're significantly increasing the time it takes to react and contributing thereby to the freeze response, but the reality is much different. Having choices gives us the freedom to weigh each option and evaluate how the outcome of that option would affect our safety. We weight these decisions well in advance of being faced with danger. That's what situational awareness is all about. Once we have a good idea of what could go wrong, and what our reactions to those events would be, choosing the appropriate solution takes only milliseconds. Options give us confidence, and that's precisely what we want for our children: for them to be confident.

When it comes to situational awareness and spotting danger, children need to understand that they have multiple options that can keep them safe. Communication, avoidance, escape, and confrontation are all valid choices, but picking the most appropriate response can be tricky for younger children. The skills they've learned up to this point will assist them in identifying the key environmental elements that aid in keeping them safe. Now let's take a look at the response options I've listed above and how each one fits into the spectrum of planning and personal safety.

6.1 Communication

Communication skills are one of the most important abilities your child can develop. Being a good communicator will serve them well in every aspect of their life all the way through to adulthood. When it comes to children and the way they apply communication to escaping danger, I don't recommend trying to teach them to negotiate with an aggressor. For children, communication comes into play when an adult needs to be alerted to the presence of a threat. Let's say, for instance, that a child becomes separated from Mom or Dad. At this point, the child's memory should be developed enough to relay to an adult the last known position of the parent, their first and last name, and what they were wearing. If that's not enough, they should also have a phone number memorized as well as the name of a trusted relative or neighbor. I know how important it is for your child to have this information memorized because, as much as I hate to admit it, I once lost my son in a crowd so large that I had no idea how I was going to find him. I know first-hand that it can happen to anyone, no matter what your level of awareness may be, and it can happen within a matter of seconds.

It happened back in 2005. My son Joshua was eleven years old and had expressed an interest in running a 5K. At the time, I was doing a lot of distance running, and I was happy that my son wanted to join in. We registered for the Susan G. Komen Race for the Cure in Las Vegas, where we were living at the time. The race started on Freemont Street and continued snaking through the streets of North Vegas for 3.1 miles. The morning of the race, my son and I picked up our race packets, and I was beaming when I helped him pin his number on his first race shirt. The streets were packed with thousands of participants, and people were jostling for a position near the starting line. As we moved through the crowd, I respected my son's budding masculinity and didn't insist on holding his hand, but I stayed right behind him as close as I could. At one point (as most racers do), he wanted to hit the bathroom before the start. I smiled knowingly and started looking around for any sign of a porta-john. I took my eyes off of my son for a split second, and when I looked down, he was gone. I was horrified! I immediately began scanning the area. Josh has red hair, so he should have been easy to spot, but I saw no sign of him. I called his name several times, but it was almost impossible to hear over the din of the crowd and the music blasting from a set of nearby speakers. I saw two possibilities: maybe he saw a porta-john and started moving in that direction, or maybe he continued moving with the crowd toward the starting line. I found some high ground on a nearby platform and began scanning the area near the toilets and the starting line. I spotted some local law enforcement officers nearby and knew that they had radios. I saw no sign of my son, so I made my way to the officers. As I was telling them what had happened and began giving them the name and description of my son, I saw a sight that I almost wrote off as a fear-induced hallucination ... there was my son walking up to the announcer's platform twenty yards away with a lady in a long flower-patterned dress and Ronald McDonald. Yes, that Ronald McDonald. Luckily, the iconic fast food clown was there as part of a race-day promotion. After sprinting to the platform and collecting my boy, I shook the clown's hand and thanked him for helping Josh. "No problem," he said, "that's one smart boy you have there." The whole thing had only lasted three minutes, but to me, it felt like an eternity. After I was able to speak with Josh about what had happened, he told me that once he realized we were separated, he had done exactly what his mom had told him to do and started looking for a woman who looked like a mother. That's when he spotted the lady in the flowery dress. She had three children with her, and Josh considered her safe to approach with his problem. The lady was more than happy to help, and as they approached the announcer's stand, Ronald McDonald had stepped in to assist. Josh had already given my full name, my description, and his home phone number to the clown, who was preparing to make an announcement over the loudspeaker when I spotted them. Shortly after that, the race began. Josh and I ran the whole course together, and he had one of the best times in his age group. I was so proud of my boy! Not just for putting everything he had into the race, but for not giving in to panic but acting in a manner that reflected the lessons he'd been given. He stayed calm, remembered what he had been taught, developed a plan, and put that plan into action. We ended up having a great time that day. The real trouble came later on when we got home. Josh couldn't wait to tell his mom how everything had gone. "How was the race, baby?" "It was great, Mom! I did really good, but Dad lost me, and Ronald McDonald saved my life ..." I had some explaining to do.

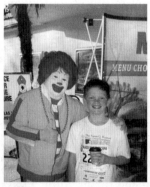

Josh and Ronald McDonald.

I look back on that story with mixed feelings. I still remember the fear I experienced in knowing I had lost track of my son, but I also look back on it with pride in knowing that my wife and I had taught him exactly what he needed to know. We all like to think that we'd never let something like that happen, but it happens regardless. I consider myself to be a good parent, and I've gone out of my way to teach my children how to be situationally aware for this very reason. We can't anticipate everything that will happen; the more variables you add (large crowds, loud music, limited visibility), the harder everything is to manage. That's why it's so important that we relinquish some of that control to our children. It does no good to have one person panicked while the other is working toward a specific goal. Teaching them how to stay calm, identify solutions, and communicate effectively with others is the best way to ensure that they're working toward the same objective you are: their complete safety and security.

6.2 Avoidance

When it comes to dangerous situations, complete avoidance is the best way to stay 100-percent safe. This is especially true for children. As we mentioned earlier, they haven't had the opportunity to develop some of the defenses we adults have. For both children and adults, being 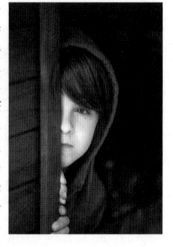 able to accurately read an area, antici- pate a dangerous situation, and remove themselves from it altogether is always the best bet. At this point, your child should have a good idea of what consti- tutes normal behavior in a variety of environments and be able to spot possi- ble threats to their safety. They should also understand their intuition and be able to articulate their feelings about various people, places, and things. Your child's ability to preemptively spot dan- gerous situations will vary depending on their age, cognitive development, and progress in their situational awareness training. Even if you're just getting started in this process and aren't quite sure how well your young one will do on their own, there are ways to help them out in terms of avoidance. Here are a couple of avoidance tactics that can go a long way in keeping your child safe.

- Designate "no go" zones. Identify areas that could pose a danger to your child's safety and let them know that these places are "no go" zones. This could include areas such as Dad's garage, where heavy tools and sharp objects pose a risk of injury; bad parts of the neighborhood; or potentially dangerous routes they may walk to and from school

- Regardless of your child's skill level, always encourage them to remain alert when they're outside or in public. This will at least get their head up and make them look like a harder target to any potential predators.

- Distance is your friend. For a predator to attack, they need three things: means, intent, and opportunity. If you take any of these three elements away, you seriously decrease their chances of success. Your child may not be able to do much about the means or the intent, but they can do something about the opportunities they present. By teaching your child to practice safe distancing from possible threats, you're effectively taking away the opportunity from anyone who may be up to no good.

If your child is a little more developed, it's easier to explain to them how all of this information begins to tie together. They start to realize that the skills they've gained through memorization, games, and role-playing are all working together toward a specific goal. You, the parent, have to make sure they fully understand what that goal is, to spot dangerous circumstances early, and avoid the situations that could pose a threat to their safety. Once my children were around ten years old, I found that they were fully capable of pointing things out that concerned them and clearly articulate why they felt the way they did. This is the point where training in evasion techniques can become more focused.

If you're practicing situational awareness and fully understand its implications, you see that staying away from danger is the best way to protect yourself from it. Once your child starts to show some level of independence, they need to understand this fact as well. Later on, we'll discuss topics such as escape and confrontation. Those are very important topics, but if you reach either of those points, something has either materialized unexpectedly, or some critical piece of information has been missed. We can't always spot every little detail that may indicate danger, but we can come close. Now, let's take a look at how everything up to this point helps with evading dangerous situations.

Think back to the skills children build through gameplay. Simple things like memorization, pattern identification, and planning all assist with awareness and avoidance. Now the games you play with your child can be more specific. When you take your child out, you can ask them more focused questions about what they're seeing. How many exits are there? Where is the nearest one? Is there anyone near us that raises your suspicion, and if so, what would you do to avoid that person if I wasn't here? Are there people near us who could possibly help you? These are the types of questions that will keep your child focused on the end goal: avoidance and therefore safety. By frequently engaging in these question-and-answer sessions, you're keeping your child dialed into their surroundings and thinking critically about the best ways to protect themselves. The more they do this, the more it starts to become second nature. It's crucial that you begin this process before their teenage years so that when they start to seek more independence, they're capable of working their way through things on their own. Teenagers tend to be more defiant, so waiting until they're older to start these discussions isn't always a good idea.

6.3 Escape

This is where things could possibly start getting scary for a child, especially younger children. Still, it's important to cover this topic. When it comes to escape, space is always a child's best friend. As I mentioned earlier, when complete avoidance of a situation is impossible, distance removes the attacker's opportunity to do harm. It's unrealistic to assume that you can keep a safe distance from everyone all the time, and this is where situational awareness aids in the process of elimination. If your child is in an area they consider to be secure, and they're surrounded by family and friends, then there's little need for them to concern themselves with distancing. If, however, they're in an unfamiliar setting populated by strangers, then maintaining a safe distance is a prudent measure. This can allow them valuable time to spot and react to potential danger. Aside from adhering to safe personal spacing, there are several other options you should teach your child to consider when making an escape.

- Is there anything you can use to divert the attacker's attention from you?
- Is there any way to create an obstacle between you and the attacker?
- Were there any safe spaces you spotted in the area that you could retreat to?
- Are there any items nearby you can use against the attacker to create space?

These are just a few possibilities when it comes to making a getaway. Always remember that there is no substitute for sound awareness and planning. Teach your child to pay close attention to their surroundings and always take note of the things that could help them make an escape if necessary, such as the number of exits and their whereabouts, the location of the closest "good guy," and any means of drawing attention to themselves that would deter a potential attacker. Remember, we're not teaching fear; do your best to keep the conversation light. If your child shows signs of uneasiness or stress while discussing these issues, back away from the subject and go 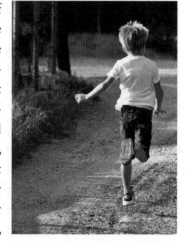 back to the more innocuous awareness exercises like games. Our goal is to keep children engaged and learning. It may seem like a lot to consider, but the more you practice and talk through these subjects with your child, the easier it gets.

6.4 Confrontation

Thankfully, the chances of your child getting into a life-or-death confrontation with an adult are extremely rare, but I've never been one to gamble with my children's safety. Think about the number of times you've been out in public and have seen a child struggling in the arms of an adult. Children are sometimes prone to tantrums, and all parents have different ways of correcting their kids in public. We witness this scenario all the time and walk right past it without a second thought. We simply write it off as a frustrated parent dealing with an unruly child. In the majority of cases, that's exactly what it is. But what if what we're seeing is something else entirely? How would we, as adults, be able to tell the difference and come to the child's aid if need be? This is why we need to broach the subject of confrontation with our children and teach them that in the event a stranger is attacking them, it's okay to 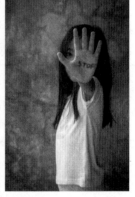 make a scene. Teach your child to scream things like, "I don't know you!" "Get away from me!" "This person is a stranger, help me!" or anything to draw attention to the situation and dissuade the attacker. Some predators can be very committed to their cause, so teach your child that in this type of situation, all manners go out the window. Let them know that it's okay to be as loud and destructive as they have to be to save themselves from an attacker. Punch, kick, scream, throw things, do whatever needs to be done.

All children are different, but all three of mine loved this part of their training. We had a large lifelike punching bag set up in the garage. I'd work with them on the proper way to throw a palm heal strike to the nose and how to deliver a swift kick to the groin. I'd let them scream at the top of their lungs while they attacked the bag. I encouraged them to be as aggressive as they wanted; nothing was off-limits.

They had a blast doing this type of thing, but I always made sure they understood the context. These types of actions are a last resort, and they're to be used only when you feel that you are in danger. My wife and I have always been complimented on how sweet and polite our children are, but we're very confident that they could fight their way to safety if the situation called for it.

Kids in Action

Little *Roman* Rescues His Mom

Roman is four years old. One day while playing at home, he found his mom lying unconscious on the floor. Roman quickly called emergency services, but it's how he made the call that's so surprising. After seeing his mom, Roman immediately took his mother's iPhone and used her thumb to unlock it. Then he activated Siri and asked it to call the police.

Roman explained to the emergency dispatch that his mother wasn't breathing and that she was "dead." They asked for his address, which Roman was able to recite immediately. Paramedics arrived thirteen minutes later. Thanks to Roman, his mom was able to regain consciousness and was treated at the nearest hospital. The local police chief released the audio recording so that others could learn the importance of teaching children basic information such as their home address. "Hearing this call brings home the importance of teaching your young child their home address and how to call the police in an emergency situation," he said. "Knowing their home address, how to call emergency services, and being able to recognize a potentially harmful situation are all important lessons for kids to lean. It could save your life and theirs."[4]

---

4 "Mummy's Not Waking Up," https://www.dailymail.co.uk/news/article-4339384/ Boy-four-saves-mother-s-life-calling-999.html.

Exercise

Play Spot the Good Guys

Now it's time to start putting a few of these practical exercises together. Spot the Good Guys, a simple version of which I introduced you to in chapter 4, is a simple and effective way to get your children engaged with their environment and thinking defensively without even realizing it. When you walk into a room, a park, or a shopping center, have your child start to pick out the people they think could be helpful in an emergency. People like police officers, uniformed security, and store employees. Once they've picked them out, have them go a step further and identify others who may be useful, such as families with small children of their own, moms pushing baby strollers, anyone who looks like they would be willing to help out in an emergency. Then start asking more specific questions:

- Why do you think that person would be helpful?
- What type of mood do they appear to be in?
- What specifically makes you think they can be trusted?

Have them be as descriptive as possible. Then have them keep a mental inventory of those people and their last known locations. If they saw a police officer when they walked in, have them remember what they looked like and where they were. Have them relate this information back to you from time to time while you're in that area. It's important that you start these types of exercises with your children when they're young. You want this to be something they do subconsciously once they're old enough to be out on their own.

Key Points

- Help your child to understand their options

  1. Communication
  2. Avoidance and distancing
  3. Escape

  —Is there anything you can use to divert the attacker's attention from you?

  —Is there any way to create an obstacle between you and the attacker?

  —Were there any safe spaces you spotted in the area that you could retreat to?

  —Are there any items nearby you can use against the attacker to create space?

  4. Confrontation. At this point, manners go out the window. Teach your child to hit, kick, scream, and do anything in their power to draw attention to their situation.

7

Common Encounters

"The greatest gifts you can give your children are the roots of responsibility and the wings of independence."

—DENIS WAITLEY

I'M NOT THE TYPE of parent to hover over my children and overreact to
the slightest possibility of danger. There have been times I've watched
my children put themselves in difficult situations and then simply waited
to see how they decided to handle the problem. "Dad! Josh is in a tree
and can't get down!" "Well, let's just see how this plays out …" "Dad!
Emily is stuck in the trash can again!" "She got herself in there. She can
get herself out …" Don't get me wrong, I would never let my children
put themselves in a position where they could be seriously hurt, but I
think it's important to let them weigh their options and work out solutions to smaller problems on their own. It's an integral part of developing their independent spirit.

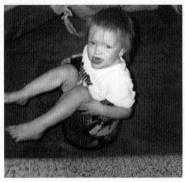

Photo by author

Emma in the trash can ... again.

As our children start to explore their independence   and create distance from Mom and Dad, they can often find themselves in situations
that frighten them. These situations can range from something as simple
as being separated from a parent in the supermarket to something as
horrific as finding themselves in the middle of a school shooting. Some
solutions are simple and others can be much more complex, but they all
require you to have a conversation with your child about how they
should be expected to react. Some reactions to problems are structured
and systematic; others are more fluid and will require some critical
thinking on your child's part. My goal here is to familiarize you with
some of the encounters your child may face and how each of these dif-
fers in terms of their response. Let's start with something simple.

- **Separation:** This is probably one of the first and most common
  frightening events that children face. Talk to any adult, and they
  will tell you a story about how they were once separated from a
  parent and how that separation caused both anxiety and fear. I
  told the story of losing my eleven-year-old son in the last chapter.
  Crowded areas like amusement parks, festivals, supermarkets,
  and malls are all rife with distractions. Your child's attention can
  be drawn away quickly, and within seconds they can find

themselves completely lost. It's important that you've trained your child in the basics before something like this ever happens. Here are a few things you should tell them before you leave the house:

✓ If you've established a meeting point, get there quickly and don't let anyone distract you.
✓ If no meeting point was established, freeze. Moving around too much could cause you to become more lost. Mommy or Daddy will come to find you.
✓ Don't be afraid to yell your parent's name. Mommy and Daddy will shout your name too.
✓ Start looking for the "good guys." If it's taking too long to find your parent, start looking for someone like an employee, security officer, or another parent who can help.
✓ Make sure you remember your parent's first and last names, as well as their phone numbers. That way, someone can make an announcement to find them.

These five simple steps can make a stressful situation much less difficult to handle. Still, you must let your child know that in the event you get separated from them, you will be working diligently to reconnect. Fear and panic can cause younger children to act erratically, which can worsen the problem.

This scenario isn't as frightening with older children. They usually have cell phones and naturally want to strike off on their own. Parents can establish preset meeting times and places to have their child "check-in" or set mandatory call times so that you know they're okay. If, for some reason, they feel that they're in danger, have them contact you or emergency services immediately.

- **Interactions with strangers:** As I've mentioned, I feel the old "stranger danger" method of handling these situations is a little counterproductive. Like my son Josh, your child may very well have to identify a complete stranger they feel is trustworthy in the event they become lost. Instead of making the hard-and-fast rule that all strangers are bad, it's best to teach your child when talking to a stranger is appropriate. When your children are with you, it's perfectly fine for them to say hello or interact with new people. You want them to be friendly and polite. Let them know you'll be right there beside them watching over the interaction. It's another matter entirely, though, if your child is alone and a stranger approaches them. Tell your child that if someone they don't know ever approaches them when they're alone and starts asking them unusual questions like, "Do you need a ride?" or "Can you help me find my puppy?" to yell, "No! I don't know you!" and leave the area immediately. Make sure they know to tell you or another trusted adult what happened as soon as possible and to remember as much about the stranger as they can. I learned while working in the federal prison system that most child predators are regular-looking people, and many go out of their way to appear friendly, safe, and approachable to children. Instead of judging a person by appearance, teach your children to judge people by their actions. It's also important to encourage kids to trust their intuition. Teach them that if someone makes them feel uncomfortable or if they feel afraid—even if they can't explain why—they need to leave the area immediately. It's not possible to protect kids from strangers all the time, but it is possible to teach them how to react and what to do if someone makes them uncomfortable.

- **School shootings:** In a perfect world, we wouldn't even need to discuss such a horrific scenario. Still, school shootings are very much a reality. Regardless of how or why they happen, your child needs to be prepared to react. In light of the increase in mass shootings, most schools have taken measures to prevent such acts, including video surveillance cameras, armed security, metal detectors, and roving patrols. Educators now routinely conduct mass shooting response drills and get certified in programs like ALICE (see below) to standardize how children should react. If you've ever found yourself in the middle of a violent encounter, one where someone is dead set on causing harm, you understand that most plans never survive first contact. Don't get me wrong, plans are a critical element of mission success, but in situations like these, it's also crucial that your child be able to think critically and be capable of deviating from the plan if circumstances call for it. Make sure your child is fully aware of the end goal in situations like these: avoid the shooter at all costs and escape to safety. I think the ALICE program is a great starting point, so let's take a look at what that plan involves. ALICE stands for:

Alert: This is when you first become aware of a threat. The sooner you understand you're in danger, the sooner you can save yourself. A speedy response is critical. Seconds count. Alert is overcoming denial, recognizing the signs of danger, and receiving notifications about the threat from others. Alerts should be accepted, taken seriously, and help you make survival decisions based on your circumstances.

Lockdown: If evacuation is not a safe option, barricade entry points into your room to create a semi-secure starting point. Use cell phones to call 911 and start preparing strategies for counter-attacking or evacuation.

Inform: Communicate information as close to real-time as possible, if it is safe to do so. Armed intruder situations are unpredictable and evolve quickly, which means that ongoing, real-time information is key to making effective survival decisions. Information should always be clear, direct, and in plain language.

Counter: Actively confronting a violent intruder is never the best method for ensuring the safety of those involved. Counter is a strategy of last resort. Counter focuses on actions that create noise, movement, distance, and distraction with the intent of reducing the shooter's ability to shoot accurately.

Evacuate: Evacuating to a safe area takes people out of harm's way and hopefully prevents civilians from having to come into any contact with the shooter.

Regardless of what program your schools have implemented, make sure that your children understand the importance of listening and communicating. Most young children are ill-equipped to deal with the stresses of such a terrifying encounter. They will look to the adults around them for support and guidance. Talk to your local school officials and become familiar with the plans they have in place. Once you understand those plans, it will be much easier to talk to your children about their responses and what they can expect from those around them. Preparation is the key to success.

These are just a few situations your child may someday face. No one can predict every threat with 100-percent accuracy, but notice that every scenario I listed has a common element—pre-planning. Carefully consider the daily routine of your children. At what points during the day could they possibly be exposed to some external threat? What is the extent of that threat, and how would you expect your child to respond? Think these things through and make sure you have a plan for how you'd like these situations resolved. Then talk to your children openly about the dangers they may face. Ask them questions about how they may react. I call this the "what if" game and I cover it extensively in my first book. This is a game I used to play with my children regularly. It ties the whole program of awareness together and allows your young one to think critically about their situation and come up with various ways to handle it on their own. Make sure you cover every aspect of their plan and that you clearly communicate the way you'd like to see the situation resolved. The outcomes are unlimited, but keep your child focused on the main objective—their complete and total safety.

Kids in Action

C. J. Saulsgiver Performs CPR

Local health officials are calling sixth-grader C. J. Saulsgiver a hero after he performed CPR on his mother, who collapsed from a heart attack. If it weren't for his actions, they said, his mother probably wouldn't be alive today. C. J. arrived home from school with a friend and had headed to the basement to hang out when he heard his mother, fifty-five-year-old Christine, call his name from upstairs. "She was upstairs cleaning, and when I got up there, her face was bright purple, and her hands were really big," said C. J.. "Then she collapsed and wasn't breathing, so I called 911." The local dispatcher told C. J. he would have to be walked through CPR, but the boy said he already knew the procedure. Three months previously, C. J. went with his parents to a CPR training course and received certification. "We were in the process of taking in a foster child, and in order to do that, you have to have CPR training," said C. J.'s father. "My wife and I were just going to go, but C. J. decided he probably should go and learn, too." When his mother collapsed, C. J. and his friend Carter rolled her onto her back. While Carter held her hand, C. J. started chest compressions and rescue breaths. "I put the phone on speaker and set it down on the floor while I did CPR on my mom," C. J. said. "I did four compressions and a breath, and she started to breathe. Then I waited a second, and she stopped breathing, so I did it again, and she started to breathe again." Christine had suffered a global heart attack, meaning the coronary vessels were blocked entirely, starving the heart of oxygen. "A good outcome from that type of heart attack is very rare," said local fire chief Jason Poulsen. "C. J. is a true hero. He did a great job of keeping his mother alive while help was on the way. If it weren't for him, his mother probably would not be alive." While in the hospital, C. J.'s mom said she has no memory of what happened. "I'm very proud of C. J. in so many ways. He's very mature for his age, and he means the world to me." At a news conference shortly after the incident, Poulsen presented C. J. with a firefighter badge, T-shirt, and plaque for his heroic efforts.[5]

Exercise

Observational Scavenger Hunt

Everyone loves a scavenger hunt, so why not turn it into a fun game that can help to build your child's situational awareness? You can do this in almost any environment. Before you leave the house, come up with a list of items that you need your child to identify. Things like a mailbox, a red truck, a woman in a dress, a small dog, or a police officer. As you walk along, your child will be on the lookout for these items. Once they spot one, mark it off the list then add another item. If you have multiple children, see who can find the most items on the list, or who finds them all first. These things can be as straightforward or as complicated as you'd like depending on the age and attention span of your child. This is a fun way to engage your kids with their environment and keep them paying attention to their surroundings.

---

5 "Utah 12-Year-Old Saves His Mother's Life with CPR," https://archive. sltrib.com/article.php?id=56047167&itype=cmsid.

Key Points

Talk to your children about some of the common emergencies they may encounter:

- Separation

—If you've established a meeting point, tell your child to get there quickly and don't let anyone distract them.

—If no meeting point was established, tell them to freeze. Moving around too much could cause them to become more lost. Tell them Mommy or Daddy will come to find them.

—Make sure they are not afraid to yell their parent's name. Mommy and Daddy will shout their name too.

—Tell them start looking for the "good guys." If it's taking too long to find their parents, they should start looking for someone like an employee, security officer, or another parent who can help.

—Make sure they remember their parent's first and last names, as well as their phone numbers. That way, someone can make an announcement to find them.

- Interaction with strangers

—Remind them that not all strangers are bad.

—Tell them to listen to their intuition when dealing with people they don't know.

- Random acts of violence/school shootings

—Make sure they know their school's plan of action for emergencies.

8

The What-if Game——Putting It All Together

"If you are truly serious about preparing your child for the future,
don't teach him to subtract, teach him to deduct."
—FRAN LEBOWITZ

AT THIS POINT, you may be asking yourself, "Now that I have all of this knowledge regarding situational awareness training, how do I put all of the pieces together to gauge what my child has learned?" I've always found that the best way to evaluate children's progress is to test them with the what-if game I mentioned earlier. After the incident at my kid's school, I seriously stepped up the amount of time I spent with them on the subject of situational awareness. As we've discussed, I felt it was important to keep the topics light and make the learning fun, but I wanted to impress upon them the importance of what they were learning and why. Once in a while, when I found a news story I thought would be of particular interest to the kids, I would share it with them, and we would work through what their responses should be if they ever found themselves in a similar situation. Due to the violent nature of some of these events, I held off on discussing them with my children until I felt they were capable of processing the information maturely. Here's an example.

On July 20, 2012, a deranged killer entered the Century 16 theatre in an Aurora, Colorado shopping mall. Within minutes he killed twelve people and injured seventy others. Back in 2012, well after the incident at the school, my three children were in their teens, and like most families with teenagers, we spent a lot of time at the mall. Given what I knew about these seemingly random acts of violence, I felt that it was necessary to inform my children about the appropriate responses to situations like active shooter events. As I mentioned in the last chapter, this can be a tough subject to broach, but it has to be discussed if you're serious about child safety. I found the best way to engage my children on this topic was to explain the event and then ask them questions about how they think they may respond in similar situations. "If we're in the food court and gunfire erupts to the left, where do we go, and what actions do we take?" "If we're entering a store and someone with a knife starts running toward us from the opposite end, what do we do?" The mental rehearsals provided by these what-if games were invaluable, and they helped us to better prepare for situations we wouldn't normally dream of finding ourselves in. My children are all grown now, but to this day they'll tell you that the what-if games I played with them when they were young have helped them to be more aware and focused in their adult lives. Experts often remind us that "the body will not go where the mind has not been." Regularly asking your children, "What would you do if ... ?" and then working through those situations is an effective way to raise their level of awareness and decrease the chances of them being caught off guard.

What-if games are an extremely effective way to increase situational awareness and decrease reactionary times in the event of a violent encounter. These games can be played in any environment and are most effective when you're playing with others. Here's how it's done.

Whenever you're out and about with your children, whether it be on a shopping errand, walking around the mall, or out to dinner with the family, take note of your position within your environment and ask your children questions about how they would react in certain situations. Start simply and then build on the scenario. You are only limited by your imagination. Here's how the progression works.

When you're out to dinner, ask your children this: what if someone enters through the back of the restaurant with a gun and begins shooting randomly? This question may catch them off guard, and that's okay. Being caught off guard and being able to think through to a solution is what this exercise is all about. Once you have their initial reaction to the event, start asking follow-up questions to flesh out their planned response and determine the safest solution to the problem.

- Is there an exit nearby you can use to get yourself to safety? If people are flooding through the doorway, is there another avenue of escape? Identify as many as possible and have them map out the best approach to each.
- Is there a place you can get to that would provide an appropriate place to hide? Identify as many as possible.
- If there is a break in the gunfire, is there something nearby you could use to cause a distraction? Is there an opportunity to escape? How?

Remember, you must have them think through each scenario you come up with to the most desirable conclusion, which is to escape safely.

What-if games are nothing more than another form of visualization and guided imagery. Much like the story of James Nesmeth in chapter 4, visualization techniques are what help elite athletes stay at the top of their game and maintain peak performance even when they are under tremendous amounts of pressure. When athletes visualize or imagine a successful competition, they actually stimulate the same brain regions as you do when they physically perform that same action. The what-if game is no different.

Michael Phelps is the most decorated Olympian of all time. He won twenty-eight medals in the thirty Olympic events he competed in, and twenty-three of those were gold. Bob Bowman has been Phelps's coach since Phelps was a teenager and has used mental imagery or visualization techniques as a regular part of Phelps's training program. Bowman instructed Phelps to watch a "mental videotape" of his races every day before he went to sleep and every morning as soon as he woke up. Phelps would visualize every aspect of swimming a winning race, starting from the blocks and ending in a celebration after the race was won. Bowman understands that visualization, without a doubt, helped Phelps develop the habit of always being successful.

"We figured it was best to concentrate on these tiny moments of success and build them into mental triggers ... It's more like his habits had taken over. The actual race was just another step in a pattern that started earlier that day and was nothing but victories. Winning became a natural extension," Bowman said.

Much like an athlete, these what-if games can help your children mentally prepare for the unexpected and significantly decrease their reactionary times should they find themselves confronted with violence. During such encounters, lives can be lost or saved in the blink of an eye. That's why situational awareness is so important. Having their head up and alert to their surroundings, paired with visualization, can have a significant impact on your child's ability to react properly and without hesitation.

Kids in Action

Virgil Smith Rescues His Neighbors

As Hurricane Harvey's floodwaters took over his first-floor apartment in Dickinson, Texas, thirteen-year-old Virgil Smith left his building and entered the dangerous waters to come to the aid of his neighbors. Virgil and his mother, Lisa Wallace, took shelter in a nearby neighbor's second-floor apartment after water rushed into their ground floor home. It was around 2 a.m. when young Virgil received a call from friends requesting help because they couldn't swim. "I was like, 'Man, I gotta go get them right now,'" Virgil told reporters. "I gotta go help my friends." Virgil swam back to his apartment from his neighbor's place to retrieve an air mattress his family stores for guests, and then sprang into action. "I put him, his two sisters, one baby, and his brother, and I had my other friend by the hand right here, and I set his momma and his step-dad on the air mattress," he said. With help from two other neighbors, Virgil guided the mattress and its passengers through the water to the second-floor room where his mother was waiting. But he didn't stop there—he and his team used the mattress to rescue other neighbors in need. Virgil says he even helped retrieve an elderly woman in a wheelchair. "She was like, 'Help, help!' and we were like, 'We got you,'" he said. Virgil's mother, Lisa, said her faith is what kept her confident as she watched her son maneuver through the debris-filled waters. "All I'm thinking about is I know he's able to save. He can rescue, he can swim, and I just had faith in the Lord that everything was gonna be alright," she said. Meanwhile, brave Virgil says he is just happy snakes or alligators didn't bite him during the rescue.[6]

---

6 "13-Year-Old Rescues Neighbors on Air Mattress During Harvey," https://abc13.com/13-year-old-rescues-neighbors-on-air-mattress-/2393284/.

Exercise

Play the What-If Game

The what-if game is a fantastic way to gauge your child's ability to think critically about their surroundings and develop plans of action based on what they see. So far, your child has been practicing the techniques that help them to identify key factors in their personal safety:

- The ability to recite critical information to other adults in the event of an emergency
- The general mood of the area and how that compares to their preconceived baseline
- The number and location of exits
- The number and locations of the "good guys"

Now, with all of this information on hand, it's time to put it all together. When you're out in a public area, present your child with scenarios that will make them think about how they should respond. Be sure to keep the scenarios age-appropriate and don't come up with anything that may cause undue fear or alarm. Here's an example. "You're at the park, and a stranger approaches you, asking if you can help him to track down his lost kitten. You look around for Mom or Dad, and you don't immediately see them. Based on the people and things you have available to you in the park, how should you respond?"

An appropriate answer would be:

"I'd immediately yell for Mom or Dad. If they don't answer, I will look for a 'good guy' in the area who may be able to help. If one isn't available, I would yell, 'I don't know you! Get away from me!' and run away from the stranger."

This is a perfectly acceptable answer, but make sure that your child stays focused on the end goal, which is their complete and total safety. As your children get older, you can change and add to the scenarios to make them more applicable to the situations they may find themselves in.

You can also guide their answers and point out things they may miss to help them arrive at the proper solution.

Key Points

- Use the what-if game to help your child develop plans of action during emergencies.
- Visualization paired with well-thought-out planning helps to decrease reaction times during emergencies.
- Work together to help your child think through their decisions and the pros and cons of each.
- Keep each plan simple and with the end goal of avoidance and safety in mind.

9

Working Together

"Children will listen to you after they feel listened to."
—JANE NELSEN

SITUATIONAL AWARENESS takes work. I wouldn't be where I am today without the leadership and guidance of some pretty amazing mentors. The awareness techniques I've presented to my children are based on the things I've learned during my nineteen years as a federal air marshal. Here, I've taken those lessons and broken them down into manageable, age-appropriate pieces that when placed together as a whole look no different than what I've done throughout my career. As an adult, it's up to you to make sure your children are prepared for the dangers life may present them. Predatory violence, kidnapping, and human trafficking aren't subjects we tend to discuss freely with our children, but if we expect them to be confident, independent young people, we have to work together with them as opposed to sheltering them from these realities. Children are capable of picking up on things that we're sometimes unaware of, so it's vital that we pay close attention to how we as adults engage with others. Younger children especially learn by observing others, and they hear almost everything. You may not even realize some of the things they're picking up on, but I can guarantee they're watching and listening.

Something I learned early on as a federal air marshal was how to interact with uniformed police officers in the event we made contact. I didn't wear a uniform, but I was armed pretty much all the time, both on and off duty. Undercover law enforcement officers need to understand how to communicate the fact that they're carrying a weapon in a way that doesn't cause panic or confusion during the interaction. Here's an example. Let's say I'm pulled over for speeding (it happens). I would pull safely to the side of the road, turn my hazard lights on, turn off the vehicle, turn off the radio, roll the window down, and place both hands on the steering wheel where they could be seen. Once the officer approaches, they almost always ask, "Do you have any drugs or weapons in the car?" I always answer with, "Sir (or ma'am), I have my duty weapon on me, and my credentials are in my back pocket." They usually respond with, "Who do you work for?" I tell them, and with my identity established, I'm normally sent on my way with a warning to slow down. I want to make it clear that I'm no speed demon, but I have been pulled over a few times, and as embarrassing as it may be, I've been pulled over while I've had my family in the car with me. I've never taken the time to explain to my children the intricacies of the interaction, but believe me, they were watching.

One year my wife and I decided to take the kids from Las Vegas, where I was stationed at the time, to Idaho to visit her brother's family for Thanksgiving. We left late one evening to return home. I planned on making the ten-hour drive at night while the kids were comfortably asleep in the back. As I drove through the seemingly abandoned desert, I started to let my impatience get the best of me, and I sped up ... considerably. When the blue light hit me, I looked down and saw that I was going a little over one hundred miles per hour. I figured I was getting a ticket for sure this time, so I pulled over, went through my routine, and patiently awaited my fate. I had the window down as my wife dug out the registration. The officer approached the driver's side of the car and shined the flashlight inside. I thought the kids were still asleep in the back when he asked, "Do you have any idea how fast you were going?" That's when my youngest, Emily, still in her car seat, started yelling from the back, "HE HAS A GUN!" The level of panic and escalation at that point was beyond words. The officer probably assumed I had kidnapped an entire family and quickly backed away from the car as he reached for his sidearm. I went into full explanation mode, "Sir, I'm law enforcement! It's my duty weapon!" It took what seemed like an eternity, but we finally got things worked out. I explained who I was and why I was armed. I didn't have a good excuse for the speeding, but once we all calmed down and the adrenaline stopped pumping, we both had a good laugh about the situation. I didn't end up in jail that night, but the officer did have some words of wisdom for little Emily: "Honey, I know you were just trying to help, but next time let Daddy tell the police officer about the gun, okay?" Emily smiled; we all thanked the officer and very slowly made our way back home.

I tell this story to emphasize the fact that even though you may not think your children are watching and listening, they are. They pick up on the slightest details, and they're perfectly capable of mimicking what they see you doing at the least opportune moments. That's why we must communicate effectively with our children and work with them as opposed to against them when it comes to explaining the way the world really works. We adults have to set the example when it comes to living situationally aware, and we have to make sure our children understand the importance of that lifestyle. Children can accomplish a lot, especially when they have the support and protection of a willing parent on their side. But how do we go about addressing their concerns regarding violence?

Highly publicized acts of violence, particularly in schools, often confuse and upset children who may feel like they're in danger. They're naturally going to look to adults for information and guidance on how they should react to these events. Parents can help children feel more secure by talking openly and honestly with them about their concerns. Below are a few recommendations from the National Association of School Psychologists (NASP) on how to help reassure your child when they begin to feel threatened by violence.

- Reassure children that they are safe and that schools are safe. Validate their feelings. Explain that all feelings are okay and assist them in expressing those emotions appropriately.
- Make time to talk. Let their questions be your guide as to how much information to provide. Be patient; children and youth do not always talk about their feelings readily. Watch for clues that they may want to talk—signs such as hovering around while you do the dishes or yard work.
- Keep your explanations developmentally appropriate.
- Early elementary school children need brief, simple information that should be balanced with reassurances that their school and homes are safe and that adults are there to protect them. Give simple examples of school safety like reminding children about exterior doors being locked, child monitoring efforts on the playground, and emergency drills practiced during the school day.
- Upper elementary and early middle school children will be more vocal in asking questions about whether they're indeed safe and what is being done at their school. They may need assistance in separating reality from fantasy. Discuss the efforts of school and community leaders to provide safe schools.
- Upper middle school and high school students will have strong and varying opinions about the causes of violence in schools and society. They will share concrete suggestions about how to make school safer and how to prevent tragedies in society. Emphasize the role that students have in maintaining safe schools by

following school safety guidelines (such as not providing building access to strangers, reporting strangers on campus, reporting
threats to school safety made by students or community members), communicating any personal safety concerns to school
administrators, and accessing support for emotional needs.
Remember the role that situational awareness plays in this
process and never miss an opportunity to emphasize that fact.

- Review safety procedures. This should include procedures and
safeguards at school and home. Help children identify at least
one adult at school and in the community to whom they'd go if
they feel threatened or at risk.

The NASP also suggests emphasizing the following points when discussing the topic of violence with your children.

- Schools are safe places. School staff works with parents and
public safety providers (local police and fire departments,
emergency responders, and hospitals) to keep you safe. The
school building is secure because (talk about specific school
procedures).
- We all play a role in school safety. Be observant and let an adult
know if you see or hear something that makes you feel uncomfortable, nervous, or frightened. (Again, stress the critical role
that situational awareness plays in this.)
- There is a difference between reporting, tattling, or gossiping.
You can provide valuable information that may prevent harm
either directly or anonymously by telling a trusted adult what
you know or hear.

Another thing you should consider establishing with your child is
set security protocols. In the Army, we used a system of challenge and
passwords to control entry into restricted areas. Someone would
approach an entry point or the fence line, and the guard on duty
would shout a challenge word. The person on the other side was

expected to respond with a corresponding password that would identify them as friendly. You have to consider your child's personal space as a restricted area. After the incident at my children's school, we felt that it was important to put these same security protocols in place with our kids. For example, suppose a stranger approached our kids and said something like, "Hey, I'm your Dad's friend John. He sent me to pick you up from school because he got stuck in traffic and couldn't make it. Hop in the car, and I'll take you home." In response, the kids were to issue the secret challenge word or phrase, which might be something like, "Can we go get ice cream first?" The correct answer would be, "No, the ice cream shop moved to Idaho." Something that no stranger could ever guess. If the wrong answer was given, the kids knew to get away from the car immediately and alert an adult to the situation. We've always found that these little security protocols were something fun for the kids. They fostered a sense of teamwork, and they gave us peace of mind in knowing that strangers wouldn't be able to approach our children easily.

These are sound suggestions that emphasize the necessity of working together to help your child feel safe and express their concerns about violence. Situational awareness is essential to your child's safety, but you can't just force-feed them this information without listening to their questions and concerns. When you start this program with your child, take the time to ask them questions and make sure they comprehend the significance of each point you're making. The only way to be certain that your child is getting the most out of these lessons is to let them know that you're working as a team. There's no obstacle that they can't overcome when they know they have you in their corner.

Kids in Action

Lexi Shymanski Saves the Day

While driving along a cliffside road, Lexi Shymanski's mother accidentally fell asleep. She veered off the road and ran the car down a forty-foot embankment, crashing it into a tree. The accident left Lexi's mom unconscious, and her baby brother Peter badly hurt. Five-year-old Lexi woke up, still in her car seat. She saw that her mom was slumped over the steering wheel and unresponsive. In that instant, little Lexi knew she had to do something to get them all out of danger. Lexi realized that their car couldn't be seen from the roadside but she knew she needed to get help. Somehow she managed to escape from the vehicle and climb up the embankment in her bare feet. Upon reaching the road, she flagged down a passing car. Fortunately for Lexi, the first driver who stopped to help was a paramedic. He quickly made his way down the embankment, rendered aid, and called for medical assistance. Lexi, her mom, and little brother were airlifted to a hospital, where baby Peter was treated for swelling in the brain, Lexi for minor injuries, and mom for multiple fractures, broken ribs, and liver damage. If Lexi hadn't acted fast like she did, both her mom and brother would have been left paralyzed, or worse. "It's crazy. I can only remember one or two times where she got out of her five-point harness previously. She somehow got out, adrenaline or whatever," Lexi's mom told local reporters. It was later revealed that medics and firefighters had to use ropes to maneuver on the embankment, while Lexi did it completely barefoot. In the face of such accidents, it's daunting to act bravely. However, little Lexi has accomplished the seemingly impossible through sheer determination and love.[7]

---

7 "Hero Canadian Girl, 5, Saves Family after Car Crash by Hiking Barefoot Up Cliff for Help," https://www.nydailynews.com/news/world/girl-5-saves-family-crash-hiking-barefoot-article-1.2315440.

Exercise

This one is simple. Pick three exercises that you and your child both enjoy and work them into a weekly schedule. Choose any of the practical exercises I've listed or one that you've come up with on your own and put it on paper. Here's an example.

Monday: One hour of adjective flash cards to build your child's descriptive vocabulary.

Wednesday: One hour of KIM's Games to develop your child's visual recall.

Friday: Family game night. No time limit. Just pick a game that helps with memory, critical thinking, strategy, planning, or deductive reasoning. Turn the phones and television off and have a good time.

What's important is that you're fostering a sense of teamwork. It's critical that your child knows you are on this journey with them. Aside from the weekly schedule (which is flexible, of course), take walks, play games, and ask questions, not only about what your child sees and hears but also about how they feel. Have them point out the things that bother them or make them anxious. Talk through the things that worry them about school, the bus ride home, or when they find themselves alone. Not only does this help to develop their communication skills, it will also let them know that you are genuinely concerned about how they are doing and that they can depend on you to help them through difficult situations. Trust is a key element when it comes to building situational awareness in young people, so find the time to work together.

Key Points

• Make sure to reinforce the following with your children:

1. Schools are safe places. School staff works with parents and public safety providers (local police and fire departments, emergency responders, hospitals) to keep you safe.
2. We all play a role in school safety. Be observant and let an adult know if you see or hear something that makes you feel uncomfortable, nervous, or frightened.
3. Reporting is not the same as tattling or gossiping. You can provide valuable information that may prevent harm either directly or anonymously by telling a trusted adult what you know or hear.

• Establish security protocols to help your child feel more secure with the adults they may interact with.

Conclusion

"There are two gifts you should give your children,
one is roots, and the other is wings."
—UNKNOWN

THERE COMES A TIME in every parent's life when you recognize you're no longer the center of your child's world. It's a harsh realization, but the joy of watching children grow and become their own person is a very gratifying experience. You know you've poured your heart and soul into raising them right, and watching them as they begin to find their individuality is part of the reward. When children enter into their teens, they feel that pull toward independence on an almost biological level. We parents can't compete against mother nature, but we can let them strike out on their own, knowing that we've given them the tools they need to be safe, secure, and confident. The self-reliance and confident spirit my wife and I instilled in our three children has led each of them into careers in the military. Joshua, my little race buddy, is now in the Army and preparing for ranger school. Elda the defender is in the Air Force and recently returned from her first deployment. Little Emily, whose skill in communication almost got me shot, is now a linguist in the Navy. I couldn't possibly be prouder of them. My greatest hope is that the techniques I've outlined in this book help your children along that path to independence as well. Just as children deserve to seek their own way, parents also deserve the peace of mind that comes with knowing they've done everything they can to raise their child's awareness of the dangers that surround them. I encourage anyone with children in their lives, be it sons, daughters, nieces, or nephews, to study the concepts and techniques I've outlined in this book and to seek as much information as possible on the subject of situational awareness. This is just the beginning. Your child is capable of learning and growing well beyond the pages of any book. Always find a way to engage with your children and keep them invested in their own safety. Let them know that you're willing to trust them as they make the journey to freedom and that you are always there to support them. Come back to these topics often and as new dangers present themselves, don't be afraid to address them head-on—just make sure you're doing it together.

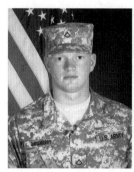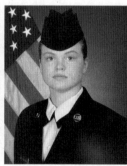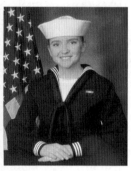

Photos provided by author

My race buddy Josh, Elda the defender, and Emily the communications specialist.

Appendix: Checklist ☑

The Roadmap to Situational Awareness for Children

The following checklist is intended to serve as a road map to help guide you along your child's journey to situational awareness and personal safety. Use it to ensure that both you and your child are meeting the standards of each of the three learning phases. Once you can confidently check each item in the first phase, you can move on to the next. This foundation of situational awareness is the most critical element in your child's future safety. Reexamine this checklist often and always take the time to revisit the basics.

PHASE ONE: The Parent's Role in Understanding Situational Awareness

☐ Develop your understanding of the reactionary gap, the OODA loop, and intuition.

☐ Comprehend various situations by establishing a baseline of behavior.

☐ Learn to spot anomalies within the established baseline through observation.

☐ Pay attention to intuition. If a situation feels wrong, find ways to get out of it.

☐ Learn to spot danger signs and pre-incident indicators:

- Hidden hands
- Inexplicable presence
- Target glancing
- The sudden change of movement

- Inappropriate clothing
- Seeking a position of advantage
- Impeding your movement
- Unsolicited attempts at conversation

☐ Study the physiological signs of danger:

- Heavier-than-usual breathing
- Appearing tense
- Pupil dilation
- Excessive sweating

☐ Avoid teaching fear, using fear as a tool, and focus lock on technology.

☐ Help your child manage their fears:

- Take your child's fear seriously
- Work together
- Give your child control
- Don't use fear as a tool

☐ Study the three primary learning mediums:

- Visual (seeing)
- Auditory (hearing)
- Tactile (doing)

☐ Use the EDIP method when teaching your child a new task:

- Explain: Give some background information on the topic and why it's important. Keep it short and simple so as not to confuse or distract anyone. Continue to explain as you carry on to the next step.
- Demonstrate: You should demonstrate what you're teaching. Make sure your child can easily see and hear you. Avoid long explanations and pauses during the

demonstration so your child can focus on observing the entire technique.

• Imitate: Get your child to imitate the methods you're teaching by mirroring you. That way, they can better understand its execution. Break things down into several sequences for easier learning if necessary. Give the feedback and correction needed.

• Practice: Get your child to practice the techniques. Note that it would not be reasonable to demand a high level of skill at this stage, as this would take more practice and time. Continue to give corrective and affirming feedback to encourage children to continue practicing.

PHASE TWO: Establishing a Foundation for Awareness

☐ Teach your children basic information they can easily relate to another adult during emergencies:

- Home address
- Parents' phone number
- Mom and Dad's place of work
- The name and number of a relative or trusted neighbor

☐ Breakdown situational awareness into its three essential components:

- Identification: The process of reading your environment based on the established baseline and identifying any behaviors that fall outside of that standard.
- Comprehension: The ability to quickly identify specific baseline anomalies and understand why that anomaly poses a risk to your security.
- Anticipation: The ability to visualize various possible outcomes based on the behaviors of the anomaly and

develop spontaneous plans of action based on the information gathered.

☐ Teach your children about situational awareness to get them dialed into their surroundings. This will naturally build their curiosity and increase their attention span.

☐ Play basic games to teach necessary situational awareness skills such as:

- Spatial awareness
- Problem-solving skills
- Analytical thinking
- Decision-making

PHASE THREE: Teaching and Reinforcing the Specific Aspects of Situational Awareness

☐ Help your child to understand and identify normal behaviors within their environment.

☐ Point out the things that concern you and have them point out the things they feel are abnormal behaviors.

☐ Use simple games and visualization techniques to help your child develop a plan of action.

☐ Teach your child that not every situation is dangerous. Make sure they understand what is and what isn't an emergency.

☐ Help your child to understand their options:

- Communication
- Avoidance
- Distancing
- Escape
- Confrontation

☐ Teach your children about some of the common emergencies they may encounter:

- Separation
- Interaction with strangers
- Random acts of violence

☐ Learn your child's school plan of action for emergencies.

☐ Use the what-if game to help your child develop spontaneous plans of action during emergencies.

☐ Work together to help your child think through their decisions and the pros and cons of each.

☐ Keep each plan simple and make sure to bear in mind the end goal of avoidance and safety.

☐ Make sure to reinforce the following with your children:

- Safety is our foremost concern. Parents, educational staff, and public safety providers (local police and fire departments, emergency responders, hospitals) all work diligently to keep children safe.
- All of us play a role in public safety. Be observant and let an adult know if you see or hear something that makes you feel uncomfortable, nervous, or frightened.
- Reporting is not the same as tattling or gossiping. Children can provide valuable information that may prevent harm either directly or anonymously by telling a trusted adult what they know or hear.
- Establish security protocols to help your child feel more secure with the adults they may interact with.

Acknowledgements

THIS IS THE SECOND BOOK in the "Heads Up" series. Although I'm getting more comfortable with the process of writing, it would be impossible to see my thoughts on the subject of situational awareness fully realized without help from some pretty amazing people.

As always, thank you so much to everyone at YMAA Publication Center. David Ripianzi, Doran Hunter, Barbara Langley, Gene Ching, and Tim Comrie, your support and guidance has made this series something greater than I ever imagined.

I've now come to the end of what I consider to be a very colorful and adventurous career in federal law enforcement. I would be remiss if I didn't acknowledge some of the men and women I've encountered whose leadership and example have shaped me into what I am today. For the sake of security, I'll not mention the names, but you all know who you are.

To the men of 1st platoon C-3/321, the junkyard dogs: you are my brothers to the end.

To the men and women at FCI Beckley, WV, and to my Special Operations Response Team (SORT) teammates: you're a bunch of dirty Vikings, and I love you.

To the dedicated men and women of USP Atwater, CA, and again to my SORT mates: although my time with you was short, the lessons you taught me about leadership and teamwork will never be forgotten.

To the dedicated men and women of the Federal Air Marshal Service: *Invisus, Inauditus, Impavidus.* Never forget why you do what you do.

Thank you to the 2007–2010 training crew in ACY. Never in my career have I worked with a more dedicated and professional group of men and women. You taught me to teach and for that I will always be grateful.

To my lovely wife Kelly: the level of support and patience you've given me as we start this new phase in our life is nothing short of amazing.

This book especially owes a big thank you to my children, Josh, Elda, and Emily. I hope the things I've taught you have served you well. This book would have been impossible to write without you. I love you, and I'm proud of you! I also apologize in advance for any embarrassment this book may cause you.

BIBLIOGRAPHY

Books

De Becker, Gavin. *The Gift of Fear: Survival Signals That Protect Us from Violence.* New York: Dell Publishing, 1997.

De Becker, Gavin. *Protecting the Gift, Keeping Children and Teenagers Safe (and Parents Sane).* New York: Dell Publishing, 1999.

Miller, Rory. *Meditations on Violence: A Comparison of Martial Arts Training and Real World Violence.* Wolfeboro, NH: YMAA Publication Center, Inc., 2008.

Web Articles and Videos

Cooper's Colors

Fairburn, Richard. "Coopers Colors: A Simple System for Situational Awareness." PoliceOne .com. Updated July 21, 2017. https://www.policeone.com/police-trainers/articles/2188253-Coopers-colors-A-simple-system-for-situational-awareness/.

Hick's Law

APA Dictionary of Psychology. "Hick's Law." https://dictionary.apa.org/hicks-law

OODA Loop

Hightower, Tracy A. "Boyd's OODA Loop and How We Use It." TacticalResponse. https://www.tacticalresponse.com/blogs/library/18649427-boyd-s-o-o-d-a-loop-and-how-we-use-it.

Family fun in a box

https://psychcentral.com/lib/family-fun-in-a-box/.

Growing independence

https://www.healthychildren.org/English/ages-stages/preschool/
Pages/Growing-Independence-Tips-for-Parents-of-Young-Chil-
dren.aspx.

Missing children statistics

https://www.missingkids.org/footer/media/keyfacts.

Why imaginative play is important to a child's development

https://www.telegraph.co.uk/lifestyle/family-time/
imaginative-play-benefits/.

Texting and driving accident statistics

https://www.edgarsnyder.com/car-accident/cause-of-accident/
cell-phone/cell-phone-statistics.html.

Media use by kids age zero to eight

https://www.commonsensemedia.org/sites/default/files/uploads/
research/csm_zerotoeight_fullreport_release_2.pdf.

How to keep your kids from inheriting your fears

https://www.fredericksburg.com/lifestyles/how-to-keep-your-kids-
from-inheriting-your-fears/article_bcc14fa5-f251-5eac-
961b-26edb55d6aee.html.

How to help children manage fears

https://childmind.org/article/help-children-manage-fears/.

How to recognize anxiety in children

https://councilforrelationships.org/
recognize-anxiety-in-your-children/.

EDIP Principle

http://www.strengthelements.com/articles/edip-principle.

The power of visualization

https://7mindsets.com/power-of-visualization/.

Emergency action plan: 5 simple steps kids can follow in an emergency

https://www.fatherly.com/parenting/teach-kids-emergency-plan/.

Heroic four-year-old saves mom's life by calling 911 while keeping her siblings and dogs calm

https://eve.womenworking.com/
hero-4-yo-saves-her-mother-by-calling-911-calms-her-siblings-
and-takes-care-of-dogs.

Nine killed in shooting at Omaha mall, including gunman

https://www.cnn.com/2007/US/12/05/mall.shooting/

Talking to children about violence: tips for parents and teachers

https://www.nasponline.org/resources-and-publications/resources-
and-podcasts/school-climate-safety-and-crisis/school-violence-
resources/
talking-to-children-about-violence-tips-for-parents-and-teachers
http://stew.ucdavis.edu/Shared_Resources/Shared_Resources_
Online/Delivery/Teaching_Methods/

INDEX

About the Author

GARY QUESENBERRY was born in the Blue Ridge Mountains of Virginia. His love of the outdoors and patriotic spirit led him to enlist in the United States Army where he served as an artilleryman during Operation Desert Storm. Gary later became a career Federal Air Marshal where he devoted his life to studying violence and predatory behavior. Now Gary has retired from federal service and serves as the CEO of 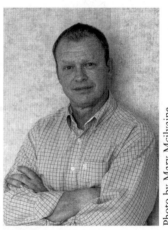 Quesenberry Personal Defense Training LLC. There he's developed numerous basic and advanced level training courses focused on mental toughness, and defensive tactics. He has an extensive background in domestic and foreign counterterror training and has worked in both the private and corporate sectors to help educate others on the importance of situational awareness and personal safety. He once again resides in his hometown in Carroll County, Virginia.

Photo by Mary Mcilvaine

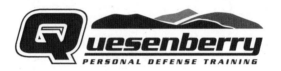

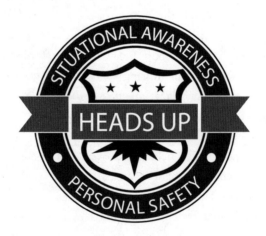

www.garyquesenberry.com

BOOKS FROM YMAA

VIDEO FROM YMAA

more products available from . . .

YMAA Publication Center, Inc. 楊氏東方文化出版中心

1-800-669-8892 • info@ymaa.com • www.ymaa.com